Animal Friendships

Research into social behavior in adult animals has often focused on aggression, yet members of social species are far more likely to interact with each other in a positive way. *Animal Friendships* explores non-sexual bonding behaviors in a range of mammals and birds. Through analysis of factors that trigger and deepen friendships, Dagg uncovers a world of intricate and complex social interactions. These factors include sources of food, formation of coalitions, play-dates for infants, mutual grooming, and the apparent pleasure of simple companionship. Chapters cover different types of friendship from those between two individuals, such as male–female or parent–adult offspring friendships, to those within family groups, and even inter-species friendships. Not only does the book explore how and why friendships form, but it also showcases the ingenious field techniques used by researchers, enabling the reader to understand the scientific methodology. An invaluable read for both researchers and students studying animal social bonding.

Anne Innis Dagg holds a Ph.D. in animal behavior and is currently a Faculty Member in the Independent Studies program at the University of Waterloo. She has had extensive field experience researching the behaviors of both mammal and bird species.

Animal Friendships

ANNE INNIS DAGG
*University of Waterloo, Ontario,
Canada*

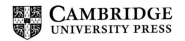

CAMBRIDGE UNIVERSITY PRESS
Cambridge, New York, Melbourne, Madrid, Cape Town,
Singapore, São Paulo, Delhi, Tokyo, Mexico City

Cambridge University Press
The Edinburgh Building, Cambridge CB2 8RU, UK

Published in the United States of America by Cambridge University Press,
New York

www.cambridge.org
Information on this title: www.cambridge.org/9781107005426

First published 2011

Printed in the United Kingdom at the University Press, Cambridge

A catalog record for this publication is available from the British Library

Library of Congress Cataloguing in Publication data
Dagg, Anne Innis.
Animal friendships / Anne Innis Dagg.
    p. cm.
ISBN 978-1-107-00542-6
1. Animal behavior. 2. Female friendship. 3. Male friendship.
I. Title.
QL751.D27   2011
591.5–dc22
                                                            2011007353

ISBN 978-1-107-00542-6 Hardback
ISBN 978-0-521-18315-4 Paperback

To Hugh, Ian, Mary, and Alan

Contents

Acknowledgments

Thank you many times to the scores of field researchers who have spent years studying the behavior of their chosen species in the wild. Without their publications, *Animal Friendships* would not have been possible. Thanks also to the following who have helped provide information for this book: Marc Bekoff, Kip Cates, Lisa Clifton-Bumpass, Pat Craton, Jean-Charles Dion, Kim Elie, Jane Forgay, Bristol Foster, Hannah Fournier, Bernice Grant, Arleen Greenwood, Lee Harding, Matt Heppler, Elizabeth Julian, Paige McNickle, Anne Miner, Colin Naga, Amy Phelps, and Paul Rose.

I am grateful also to the many friendly folk at Cambridge University Press, especially Martin Griffiths and Jeanette Mitchell with whom I worked most closely; I greatly appreciate their professionalism and empathy.

Introduction

Every day for many years I watched our three female cats, Silver, Tiger, and Gomer. Silver and Tiger were best buddies but Gomer was a loner. Actually, Silver and Tiger were half-sisters, although how would they know this? Silver, named by my young daughter Mary (although the cat was black with a white throat patch) came first, as a kitten given to our family of five by friends who had a sexually too-active female. A year later they gave us Tiger, with gray tabby markings, also as a kitten. Silver cuddled and licked her new young friend as they snuggled together. But when full-grown, both ignored the calico cat Gomer who arrived at our house as an older adult. Gomer retaliated by hissing and striking out at them with her paws. Did Silver and Tiger know somehow that they were related, which cemented their lifelong bond? Was it because Tiger came as a kitten whom Silver could mother, while Gomer (also known fittingly as Crosspatch) did not? Is it impossible for cats to become friends as adults, even though they live for years together in the same house?

Because these cats daily reminded me that animal friendships have been under-studied and under-reported, I decided to make this my next book's topic: not alliances involving youngsters that are highly instinctual – mothers and their nursing young or siblings growing up together; not matings between males and females that are short-term; but friendships between adult individuals in the wild, perhaps for evolutionary reasons or just because a duo has bonded and wants to spend much time together relaxing, feeding side by side, or grooming each other – and not all animals either, as at present we know little about the sensibilities of cold-blooded species. However, there is recent proof that three-spined stickleback fish recognize by olfaction and like to hang out with individuals from their own neighborhood (Ward *et al.*, 2007), that lizards kept as pets can distinguish between different human family members (Lee Harding, personal communication, 2010), and that dominant male hissing cockroaches from Madagascar defend a territory against other males within which they court several females who are free to come and go as they wish (Bullington, no date). Perhaps in a few decades, after far more research has been done, we will have to acknowledge that, like birds and mammals, individuals of cold-blooded vertebrates and invertebrates can also have sophisticated social systems and special friendships.

I hope this book will encourage my colleagues in behavioral sciences to look more broadly and deeply into animal friendships, the better to understand the evolutionary basis of sociality in general. In addition, a book about friendships of mammals and birds, particularly special bonds between duos, should appeal not only to scholars of animal behavior (because all the information it contains is fully referenced), but also to all people who love animals and value friendship. Men and women have adult friends for a variety of reasons: they had been early playmates, school or university chums, workmates, relatives, and/or had mutual experiences such as arise from being in the military, enduring long-term hospital stays, or sharing hobbies or common interests. Our human friends are familiar to us and compatible. (We must except, in general, "friends" featured on Facebook and MySpace who are not necessarily good friends at all and are, on occasion, forcibly "unfriended" by being removed from a site.)

There are three reasons why preferred friendships may not be present, or at least cannot be detected in a species. One is that the animals in a group are *so* closely bonded together that it is impossible to detect extra-friendly couples. Such animals are elephants and orcas (killer whales), both species considered in the chapter: *Family and group tight bonds*. The second is that many species live solitary rather than social lives, such as leopards, cheetahs, cougars, duikers, okapi, and orangutans.[1] The third category includes social species, but not social in a way that seems to need or allow special friendships to develop; the subject of the chapter: *Social but seldom sociable animals*.

What about individuals who like to stay close together? We may not know exactly what friendship means to them, or why they favor one individual above another, but in any case, it is a pleasure to know, write, and read about the caring intimacy of chimpanzee mother and grown daughter Flo and Fifi; the camaraderie of male baboons Boz and Alexander who spent much time greeting each other every morning and fighting each other's battles; and the easy companionship of Baggage and Mrs Brown, the female hyena pair in the Ngorongoro Crater who raised their youngsters together almost like family.

STUDYING ANIMAL EMOTIONS

The idea that non-human animals have feelings as we do and may even have close friendships among themselves has a checkered history. Human beings in the Neolithic Period, who were the first to domesticate animals, would probably have agreed that animals could be friends. Farmers living close to their livestock would have seen pairs of horses who especially liked to be near and to groom each other, or pig duos who spent most of their time together while resting or rooting for food. I am sure they would have acknowledged that animals have feelings and can suffer, even as people today who have companion animals such as dogs and cats would agree. Aesop's fables, for example, from the sixth century BC, explore the similarity between animal and human emotions and behavior.

With the rise of Western modern religions, however, spiritual leaders have defined all living beings except humans as inferior, and therefore subject to any form of control that people wish to have over them. Early professional scientists took especial advantage of this bias so that they could differentiate themselves from amateurs; it was important for professionals not to be seen as anthropomorphic. René Descartes (1596–1650), for example, considered animals as machines or robots, without feelings or senses as we know them. Scientists are still taught to avoid anthropomorphizing, with any inference that non-human animals have feelings, or self-awareness, or even consciousness often challenged by peers. This has surely stifled research into non-human animal social interactions.

Disdain for animals continues to be widespread, even today, in many animal-related activities where workers, sport hunters, and fishers insist that vertebrates do not have emotions or senses like our own. They must take this stand, otherwise researchers would be forced to be far more selective when they do painful experiments on live animals (Dagg 2008); zoos would be morally unable to keep social animals in barren, small cages; circuses would have to admit that training tigers and elephants is a hurtful enterprise; hunters and fishers would not be able to consider their activities as sporting fun; and rodeo workers would be unable to rationalize the roping and torment of calves as entertainment – in 2009 at least one columnist wrote, about a rodeo, that animals do not have "feelings" and have no memory of pain imposed upon them, so that infliction of pain is acceptable (Gunter, 2009).

Early research into animal behavior took place in zoos, but results could not reflect real-life conditions. For example, Michael

Chance (1956), who studied rhesus monkey activity in the London Zoo, devised an experiment that was itself biased. For his methodology, he identified the adult males in the colony "by the letters D1, D2 and D3 etc., indicating their position in the male hierarchy. The adult females were not similarly identified, but mentioned only as and when they were observed in association with particular males." Not surprisingly, Chance concluded that the social life of these monkeys revolved around the dominant males. What other conclusion could he have made? There was little concern about what females were up to or the importance of female choice of a mating partner, even though, as early as the 1850s, Charles Darwin had thought this to be vital.[2]

In the late 1950s, zoologists interested in studying animal behavior began to leave laboratories and zoos to go overseas to carry out research. I was one of the first, observing giraffe behavior in South Africa in 1956–1957 (Dagg, 2006). Other early researchers were Japanese zoologists anxious to study the activities of chimpanzees and gorillas, our close relatives, believing that their social behavior would shed light on that of our early human ancestors (Nishida, 1990). When they realized by 1966 that the behaviors of peoples and apes were quite different, they decided to carry on research of chimpanzees anyway to learn more about "another unique species." Intense interest in our closest relatives continues, with over 40 African research sites on chimpanzees and bonobos now in existence (Stumpf, 2007).

All zoologists in the field keep copious notes and records of what animals are doing each day, but these have tended toward documentation of aggression and reproduction. From my own research on giraffe, I find it easy to understand why fights and other exciting behaviors have been more likely to be noted and recorded for a social species than the simple fact of some individuals hanging out together in a congenial fashion (Dagg, 2006). Grazing, resting, chewing their cud, and walking are the norm for giraffe, but such activities hardly seemed to me worth documenting in great detail compared to the much rarer fights, male necking sessions, and reproductive behavior. It was also difficult to tell individuals apart in that low-technological age, so early research focused on the behavior of animals by sex and age class, with interest in individual relationships flowering only later after methods of identifying individuals were perfected, whether through the recognition of natural, unique markings or physical features, or by festooning individuals with rings, bands, tags, tattoos, brands, paint, or collars.

One example relates to a large international conference on ungulate behavior I attended in 1971, where there was almost no information in the many presentations about friendly activities (Geist and Walther, 1974). Instead, researchers delved at length into such topics as feeding, maternity, courtship and reproduction, territoriality, and aggression in a wide variety of hoofed animals.

As another example, some populations that would seem ideal for the study of friendship have been largely ignored until recently. In their book *Social Structure in Farm Animals* published in 1979, authors G. J. Syme and L. A. Syme note that "Investigation of 'prosocial' behaviour, for example, is almost entirely neglected in the farm animal literature." Their index lists 96 percent more line items on information about aggression, territoriality, competition, and dominance compared to line items on social attachment, social preference, and familiarity. The authors argue the urgent need for more detailed information about social behaviors, which is slowly being addressed.

Although up until the 1960s publications touching on behavior were not based on extensive field research, there was an assumption that our early human ancestors were aggressive hunters and that aggression was central to human evolution (Dagg, 2005). After Raymond Dart discovered the first *Australopithecus* fossil in South Africa in 1924, he envisioned killer apes that slaked their "ravenous thirst with the hot blood of victims and greedily [devoured] livid writhing flesh" (Johanson, 2009). The books *African Genesis: A Personal Investigation into the Animal Origins and Nature of Man* (1961), and *The Territorial Imperative: A Personal Inquiry into the Animal Origins of Property and Nations* (1966) by Robert Ardrey, *The Naked Ape* by Desmond Morris (1967), and *The Imperial Animal* by Lionel Tiger and Robin Fox (1971) valorized our "cousins" the baboons for their supposed fierceness rather than chimpanzees (then wrongly seen as much more pacific) in our evolutionary history. The activities of females, who are virtually always more friendly than males no matter what the species, were largely ignored (Kappeler, 2000).

Nature red in tooth and claw? Actually, no. Today, sociality rather than aggression is seen as the basic behavior of our early human ancestors who evolved, because of their small size, as lowly vegetarians and scavengers, not mighty hunters (Sussman and Chapman, 2004; Hart and Sussman, 2005). In the past for monkeys and apes, the most-studied species, aggression was considered as far more important (as well as more exciting) than pacific activities. "Researchers have focused their attention on competitive and aggressive behaviors, and have tended to overlook the importance of cooperative and affiliative behaviors" (Sussman *et al.*, 2005). Robert Sussman and his colleagues (2005), after surveying 81 behavioral studies of primates involving 60 species, found that diurnal group-living prosimians, New World monkeys, Old World monkeys, and apes had an exceedingly low rate of aggressive behaviors within their communities, normally less than one percent of their activity budget. By contrast, they spent on average between 85 to 96 percent of their activity time in affiliative behavior – grooming, playing, huddling, cooperative infant care, food sharing, alliances, coordinated hunting, and defense of infants and resources. Obviously, many primatologists have been intent on studying uncommon behaviors while largely ignoring common ones.

Within the past few decades, I am glad to report, there has been a swing toward regarding non-human animals as similar to ourselves in that they not only have feelings, senses, and suffer when hurt, but they may scheme to improve their own conditions by forming coalitions and alliances with other individuals. The importance of close friendships in animals was initially showcased in 1985 by Barbara Smuts when she published *Sex and Friendship in Baboons*. This book detailed the central role that non-sexual friendships between males and females play in olive baboon (*Papio cynocephalus anubis*) society. Relationships between group members of various species, especially primates, continue to be researched and the results published. Recently too, Marc Bekoff, Jeffrey Moussaieff Masson, and Frans de Waal have all written less academic but exciting books about similar traits that have a huge audience; these men are not ashamed of being anthropomorphic, but delight to depict animals as the thinking, feeling individuals they are. An international group of primatologists, psychologists, ethicists, and other experts has founded the Great Ape Project, the aim of which is to confer basic legal rights on the great apes so that they will no longer be killed, tortured in experimentation, or held in confinement.

AGGREGATIONS AND SOCIALITY

An animal "aggregation" is a general term, indicating that many individuals of a species tend to gather together although they do not interact in any significant way. Being around others of one's own kind is obviously immensely important to many species. Why else would snow geese form flocks of 42,000 for example, and Pacific black brant flocks of 175,000 (Masson, 2003)? Why else would wildebeest and zebra in East Africa choose to migrate together in herds of tens of thousands?

A "social" group, by contrast, is one of limited size in which animals *do* interact and treat each other as the individuals they are, taking into account their age, sex, reproductive condition, and personal histories. Usually, all members of a social group are at least neutral toward each other; if a duo were enemies (as two males are most likely to be), the stronger would probably have driven the other away.

Generalities about sociality are both positive and negative, but always involve tension for group members because of the pull of his or her own inclinations against the push of group needs. Being social is beneficial because it allows individuals to be friendly rather than aggressive with each other; for herbivores, it increases the likelihood of predators being detected (and for predators, such as lions, to detect them); and it increases the number of animals who might discover resources of food and water for the benefit of all. In addition, for species in which individuals groom each other, it improves their psychic and bodily health and reduces their parasite load. Herbert Prins (1996) notes that because perfect information is hardly ever available to any one individual, sharing information such as occurs in African buffalo leads to better decisions for the group, just as it does in human beings (see the chapter: *Social but seldom sociable animals*).

Social life can be negative because of increased competition for food, water, mates, and resting or sleeping sites; a greater likelihood that disease and parasites will spread among group members; and the need to defend individual space. To counter the problem of competition over limited resources, most social species (but not olive baboon males) have dominance hierarchies to prevent constant squabbles. The most aggressive individuals become the most dominant (alpha) animals who take the best of what is on offer, while those who are subordinate give way to them and to other animals more dominant than they are. This ranking reduces fighting and therefore injuries within a group. The main benefit for a dominance hierarchy in females and their offspring is access to food resources, while that for males is access to females in estrus with whom to mate.

Sociality is so central to the lives of many species that enforced isolation for individuals may make them sick (House *et al.*, 1988). It presumably evolved because it made members of a group more reproductively successful than they would have been otherwise. It also changed them anatomically. Dorothy Cheney and Robert Seyfarth (2007) from the University of Pennsylvania argue, from their lengthy research on wild chacma baboons in Botswana, that as a consequence of social interactions, the primate brain has undergone significant enlargement and increase in complexity over time.[3] In a non-social species such as the leopard or hare, a member has only itself and perhaps its young to consider. If it can find enough to eat, water to drink, a mate with whom to copulate, and can avoid predation, it is doing well. In a social species, a member has these mandates, but also must understand social relationships among all individuals of the group, which he or she can sometimes manipulate to support his or her activities.[4] Other social species have sophisticated mental powers, too: sheep subject to experimental testing were able to recognize the faces of 50 other sheep, and remember these faces individually for over two years (Kendrick *et al.*, 2001). Michael Ghiglieri (1988) agrees that keeping track of social relationships has been important in the evolution of the primate brain, but feels that the necessity to retain information pertaining to the environment has also been vital. He notes that for chimpanzees living in the Kibale Forest of Uganda to thrive, individuals must remember the location of hundreds of fruit trees (78 percent of the diet of the Ngogo chimpanzees comes from fruit) and the random times at which each bears fruit, as they do not do so in synchrony.

ENVIRONMENTAL FACTORS AND FRIENDSHIPS

The likelihood of close bonds being present in dyads of a social species may depend in part on three external factors: food, predation, and infanticide. For social hoofed animals that spread out to browse and graze, there is always tension between the need to find forage and the compulsion to stay close enough together to keep an effective watch for predators. When herds move from site to site, they do so as a group, but they lack close bonds between individuals.

If food is "clumped," meaning that it exists in quantity in limited areas that can be defended, then social behavior is more complex:

- Individuals may form coalitions, even close bonds, to try to keep food for themselves at the expense of other group members.
- Groups may have a dominance hierarchy where the strongest individuals have first dibs on available food; however, hierarchies do not tend to foster friendships except, often, for individuals related genetically to each other.
- Lions survive on an extremely "clumped" food, meat, yet the sexes form close friendships within each pride. The females bond into a hunting sisterhood in order to bring down large game animals that could not be taken by a single lion, and the males form a close brotherhood that hopes to defeat previous pride males in battle to become members of a pride themselves.

Infanticide is an insidious factor because it may occur within a group where one might have thought one would be safe. It is difficult to research because it happens rarely (and usually not at all) depending on the species (van Noordwijk and van Schaik, 2000). Indeed, sometimes infanticide is said to occur as an evolutionary strategy, when it may not be at all.[5] Recently much research has been dedicated to the topic not only of rarely seen infanticide itself, but to the *possibility* of infanticide, which is presumed to have affected the behavior of both males and females.

The focus has been on infanticide by males, especially in primates. Theoretically, such killing indicates that the female will come into estrus sooner than otherwise and will then mate with the male to produce his young. This scenario suits the new males, but is negative for the female who has wasted her energy on progeny she has produced and nursed. Infants are deemed not vulnerable to infanticide if their mothers conceive shortly after giving birth so that the period of lactation overlaps the subsequent gestation – if she is already pregnant, there is no point in killing her infant. Nor are the infants vulnerable if breeding is seasonal; if all the females copulate each year at about the same time, then no female will be receptive again until the next season. Infants of a species are deemed vulnerable to infanticide by males if the females have no set breeding period and if their lactation period is greater than the length of gestation (van Schaik, 2000).

Here are three examples of how possible infanticide by males might have fostered friendly behaviors through evolution (Paul *et al.*, 2000):

- Females of both olive baboons and chacma baboons form sociable pairs with specific males; should a male new to the troop threaten a female's young, her male friend will help protect it (Smuts, 1985; Palombit, 2000; see the chapter: *Male and female pals – not just for sex!*). For chacma baboons at least, the male shares close genetic ties with his friend's infant, usually as its father (Huchard *et al.*, 2010).
- In multimale groups of hanuman langurs, infants are protected by males who are their genetic fathers or long-time troop residents; newcomer males do not defend infants. Statistically, rates of infanticide decline as the number of males in a group increases; when a female copulates with many males, in what is called "confusing paternity," this behavior dramatically reduces the incentive of a newly dominant male to commit infanticide (Janson and van Schaik, 2000).

- Cooperating in the handling of an infant by two males presumably helps prevent infanticide, as seemed to be the case for Tibetan macaques *Macaca thibetana* (Ogawa, 1995; see the chapter: *In brotherhood*). Infanticide is obviously reduced when males interact frequently with infants because they are likely to be present if an aggressive male tries to attack a youngster.

Infanticide by females has been an overlooked topic of research,[6] but it, too, may be responsible for the bonding of individuals. Theoretical counterstrategies to the threat of infanticide from females within the same group and from other groups include (Digby, 2000):

- mothers forming coalitions to protect their young,
- females banding together to defend a territory against females from other groups,
- females remaining in their natal troop surrounded by their lifelong buddies rather than emigrating at puberty to another group,
- females harassing immigrant females lest they harm their young, and
- dominant females suppressing reproduction of subordinate ones.

But it is impossible to know for sure if these behaviors have evolved because of the threat of infanticide.

BENEFITS OF A SPECIAL FRIENDSHIP[7]

This book is about friendship, but particularly special friendships between two or among a few individuals. How does such a friendship benefit adult animals (Cords, 1997)?

- They frequently offer egalitarian companionship.
- Friends can alert each other to danger, or a water or superior food source.
- They may share food.
- They support each other in conflict or possible infanticide.
- They may groom each other, offering sensory pleasure and the removal of dead skin and parasites.
- They can perhaps "teach" each other something new, such as sharing recent information.
- They can help reduce emotional distress.
- They can take advantage of altruistic behavior.

- If they are of unequal dominance, the higher ranked animal can be a great use to the lower one in that the latter's status (and sometimes that of its relatives) will improve.
- Primates sometimes care for their friends by such things as removing fly eggs or maggots from their festering sores (Goodall, 1986).

This list indicates that special friendships are positive for non-human animals as well as for people. It is great to have a person with whom to share news, who cares what you do and what you say, who is pleased when you have accomplished something special, and grieves with you in times of sadness. Isolation not only makes us unhappy, but is also unhealthy: it increases blood pressure, stress levels, general wear and tear on the body, and the chance of developing Alzheimer's disease. It may also hasten death (Cacioppo and Patrick, 2008). We can infer that the ability of a woman to produce up to 20 children in her lifetime is only possible because our distant ancestors had, as well as mates, close female friends who helped each other cope with offspring much nearer in age than the offspring of the great apes (Hrdy, 2009).

Despite its charms, not all animal species have friendships or a social life. Whatever lifestyle is effective for a species depends ultimately upon the environment and the way a species has adapted to it – lions hunt cooperatively to bring down large prey, while leopards prey individually on smaller species. Orangutans have been described as "hardly more social than any mammal must be," which means a mother raising her infant, and a male and female getting together for sex (Montgomery, 1991). Biruté Galdikas followed a female orangutan, Fran, for many years in the wild. Her daughter, Fern, traveled with her during her first pregnancy, but when her infant was born, she broke away from her mother and, for the next ten and a half years, the two did not associate, on occasion "just moving by each other with not so much as the blink of an eye to signal overt recognition." Then Galdikas saw the two together again in the forest canopy. After a decade of separation, the two embraced and traveled together for four days. Such solitary species are not part of this book.

WHAT CONSTITUTES A SPECIAL FRIENDSHIP?

The earliest bonds in mammals are between a mother and her newborn offspring whom she suckles; indeed, mother love may be the root of all love. Siblings usually form bonds too, as they grow and play together.

And male and female adults get together briefly to mate. But these time-limited attachments are not part of this book. Rather, I consider here two kinds of special friendships between and among adults.

The first is related to the evolution of a species, as the following examples indicate:

- Male and female geese bond together because this is the most effective way to produce young who will thrive.
- Male and female olive baboons form platonic relationships that provide protection for the female and her young.
- Lionesses develop tight bonds with other female pride members from the time of their birth which makes them great communal hunters. Male lions bond with other males to become, in time, pride males who can and have defeated other pride males.
- Friendliness has been bred into dogs over centuries to such an extent that they are usually upset if other dogs or people ignore them (Masson, 1997).

In social species, some or all of the young disperse when they are old enough to venture off on their own. This gives the emigrating individuals better mating opportunities and prevents both inbreeding and overcrowding in the natal population. There is a genetic bias toward which sex will emigrate in a species, and therefore also usually a bias toward possible friendships. In many or most species, females form the stable core of a group from which adolescent males disperse when they reach puberty (such as lions, common baboons, Japanese monkeys). The females of such a group, who have known each other since birth, are familiar and often friendly toward each other, interactions with relatives being especially positive. For species in which females leave their natal group (such as chimpanzees, hamadryas baboons, gorillas), the males sometimes retain male friendships from their youth or with their grown sons. Among primates, female–female bonds are much more common than male–male bonds because the resources that limit the reproductive success of females (food, safety) can be shared more easily than can those of males (copulations) (van Hooff and van Schaik, 1992).

The second kind of friendship is formed by individuals because of a deep affection between them. Konrad Lorenz (1952) talks about "falling in love," which indeed can happen almost instantaneously for wild geese and jackdaws, just as it does for some people. It is not only a matter of sex. Members of these two species join forces in the spring following their birth and stay together until they become sexually mature a year later when they mate and begin a family. Jeffrey Masson agrees with Lorenz, writing (1999): "Animals, like people, form deep attachments to other animals and other people, often of the same sex, for reasons that have nothing to do with genetic advantage and everything to do with emotions, and one emotion in particular: love." Both kinds of friendship last for months and even for many years.

DEDUCING FRIENDSHIPS

Anthropologist Joan Silk from the University of California in Los Angeles organized probably the first symposium on the subject of friendship in non-human animals and arranged for the publication of the presentations in the journal *Behaviour* (2002). In her introductory paper "Using the 'F'-word in primatology," she notes that those who study primate behavior have defined this word in a variety of ways. Some primatologists even deny that relatives can be true friends in that their relationship is defined instead as enlightened self-interest governed by genetics (Ghiglieri, 1988); it has been called reciprocal altruism in that individuals may perform favors for a relative with the expectation that these favors will be reciprocated at a later time (Silk, 2002). However, for most social groups of animals, we do not know who is related to whom because their relationships have not been documented over many years. Nor does such a cold-blooded concept of friendship seem suitable to my way of thinking. For this book, therefore, I shall consider two animals to be special friends if they act as if they like each other, even if we do not know why they do so (Noë, 2006). It is easier to infer friendships among mammals than among birds, in part because we ourselves, as mammals, are more attuned to beings like ourselves. Birds do not have arms or hands with which to embrace and touch each other, and mutual preening tends to be related to aggression rather than friendship (see the chapter: *Fathers and sons, and social grooming and preening*). Additionally, few birds apparently form friendships beyond those that, by instinct, impel them to be supportive of their own immediate family members. In the literature, twosomes who are very close have been denoted in various studies and species as Friends (with a capital F) for male and female olive baboons (Smuts, 1985), as SSFs (specific senior females) for female bonobos (Idani, 1991), as PPRs (peculiar-proximate relations) for male and female Japanese monkeys (Takahata, 1982), or more generally as pair-bonds (Fuentes, 2002).

We cannot ask either mammals or birds about their feelings, but it seems sensible to assume that individuals have a special friendship if they remain close together for extended periods of time (Cords, 1997). For olive baboons, Barbara Smuts (2001) notes that factors affecting whether an animal allows another into its personal space include gender, age, relative status, and especially familiarity and trust. Friends also often do the same things at the same time (*pace* petrel and albatross couples, as described in the chapters: *Male and female pals – not just for sex!* and *In sisterhood*). In general (and depending if such activities are in a species' repertoire of behaviors), signs that individuals may be special friends include not only often being together but also:

- grooming each other more than they groom anyone else (Cords, 1997),
- embracing each other (woolly spider monkey),
- vocal exchanges (gibbons),
- homosexual mountings (gorillas),
- genital contact (bonobos),
- genital touching (baboons) involving huge trust between participants,
- reciprocity between positive behavioral acts (various acts in various species).

We cannot know the precise meaning of such behaviors, of course, and there is an additional caveat: in one species that has been studied in great detail, the Japanese monkey, presumed friendships between individuals differ depending on the activity measured, in this case proximity, grooming, and vocal exchanges (see the chapter: *Male and female pals – not just for sex!*).

We can assume that friendship of some sort exists in socially monogamous species, but the friendships included in this book are held to a high standard, with a pair staying together for considerable time. In the case of a mated pair, their bond must last longer than the time they spend raising their young, and it sometimes endures for a lifetime of raising offspring sequentially. Special friendships cannot be casual ones such as occur only in short-term coalitions formed for a specific purpose.

One has to be careful in deducing friendships between individuals, however. For example:

- Tourist groups in Africa who see a male and a female lion resting companionably together might assume that they are good buddies. This is not the case (Schaller, 1972). Pride lionesses hang out together a great deal, and pride males are also bonded, but males and females are only casually interested in each other except during courtship, when the female is in estrus. At that time, relations are intense but short-lived: one female and male copulated 157 times in 55 hours. Nomad lion groups may include both males and females, but these ephemeral aggregations break up frequently, with members going their own way.

- Although some pairs of chimpanzees virtually never groom and are rarely in contact, they may be seldom more than nine meters (30 ft) apart and may defend each other in fights, which indicates a psychic friendship if not a readily apparent one (Goodall, 1986).
- Individuals may be judged to be friends because they are often seen together. However, their proximity may be misleading. They may congregate because there is food in the area or shade against the sun, or females may gather around a male they all like although they do not like each other (Nakamichi, 1991).
- When a female vervet or macaque monkey, or baboon gives birth, she becomes extremely attractive to the other females in her group even if she is of low rank; they are anxious to sit by her and groom her because they want to have a chance to groom and handle her infant (Cheney and Seyfarth, 1990). When the youngster grows older though, the mother loses her cachet and her temporary "friends."
- For Japanese monkeys, proximity behavior may mean psychic closeness, but it may also mean, in the winter mating season, that old females are trying to avoid sexual aggression from males by huddling near other animals to keep warm (Kato, 1999).

ORGANIZATION OF THIS BOOK

The information about friendships contained in this book is necessarily skewed, because animals such as apes and monkeys have been studied in endless detail while we know little about the behavior of uncommon or small social species. The chapters are devoted to each type of possible special friendships between male and female adults with the exception of males and their adult daughters; such dyads seldom exist because of the possibility of inbreeding: adolescent daughters of a male will have emigrated from their natal group to another group or the fathers themselves will have been replaced (as in lions) by the time their daughters reach adulthood. There are only a few known exceptions. In Dian Fossey's (1983) gorilla group 5, the dominant male

Beethoven mated with his daughter Pantsy to produce Banjo, but after that, refused to mate with her again; she and his son (her half-brother) Icarus then paired up. Incest has also been documented in beaver (Ryden, 1989), wolves (Ellis, 2009) chimpanzees (Goodall, 1986), and mole-rats (Clutton-Brock, 2007).

In addition to the bonded pair possibilities, the chapter: *Family and group tight bonds* deals with groups of animals where there is a close bond between three or more rather than just two; the chapter: *Old buddies* with tight pairs of old animals; the chapter: *Social but seldom sociable animals* with species whose behavior has been well researched but whose members have never developed particular friendships among themselves, and why this might be the case; the chapter: *Cross-species pals* with relationships between animals of different species (which are mostly shorter term because of their nature); and the chapter: *Animal and human "friendships"* with firm friendships between animals and people (although the term "friendship" is perhaps not applicable when the two members of the dyad do not have equality, as will be discussed in this chapter). Two topics that, in some species, may affect friendship behavior to some extent (researchers offering group members free food) or that are closely correlated with friendship (grooming) are included in the two shortest chapters: *Mothers and sons, and providing free food* and *Fathers and sons, and social grooming and preening*, respectively. There are many examples of close friendships for the three most common dyads (a male and a female, two females, two males), so I have chosen those between pairs in species that illustrate the great variety of possible relationships.

The scientific names of the species discussed in the text are those given by the researchers. Chacma baboons are sometimes called *Papio ursinus* and sometimes *Papio cynocephalus ursinus*. Similarly, the olive or anubis baboons are called either *Papio cynocephalus anubis* or *Papio anubis*.

This book reports widespread friendship among animals, a delight both in and of itself – red in tooth and claw does not begin to depict nature. It also highlights and pays tribute to the many field researchers who have spent years of their lives in the field, watching and analyzing the social behaviors of "their" species. Animal pairs held captive in zoos or circuses or subject to experimentation are, in general, not considered in this book because these are unnatural conditions to which it would be wrong to give credence.[8]

The study of animal relationships is never cut-and-dried. Even within one species, behavior is influenced by such things as race, group size, group dynamics, food supply, and habitat. Friendships may be present between different sets of dyads or groups in a species in one area, but not in another. Or anomalous friendships may occur for no apparent reason, such as the three male cheetahs who banded together to hunt prey, even though cheetahs are considered to be basically solitary (King, 2009). Further research will certainly refine what we now know about animal friendships. In addition, the new ability to analyze DNA from an individual's feces is a huge step forward in that the genetic relationships of individuals in a group can now be determined. Until recently, long-term studies were necessary to know who was related to whom maternally in a social group and paternity was always a guess (Chapais and Bélisle, 2003).

The first chapter will consider male and female friendships. Many people assume that most animal species live in couples with their young, because we do (in theory) ourselves. If they see a photograph of a male, female, and young giraffe, or of a mallard duck and drake near ducklings, they perceive each as families, although neither group merits that word. Male and female individuals, such as birds who work together to bring up their offspring, or beaver who remain housemates even when they are not raising a litter, or male baboons who become buddies to females caring for their infants, are by no means common in the entire animal kingdom.

Male and female pals – not just for sex!

We think of ourselves as a monogamous species, so it seems strange that among our closest relatives, chimpanzees, bonobos, and gorillas, males and females do not form pairs but rather consort with a variety of mating partners. Few primates know who their father is. The most devoted couples among non-human species, instead, are birds of whom over 90 percent are monogamous (Adkins-Regan and Tomaszycki, 2007) – socially monogamous, that is; recent genetic research into the DNA of nestlings proves that many species have males and females who commonly mate with individuals other than their avowed partner. The necessity for social monogamy in birds is related to reproduction, with the laying of eggs by females rather than the production of live young who nurse from their mother. The eggs have to be protected during incubation and the insatiable nestlings fed until they are able to fend for themselves. This requires a huge amount of parental effort, especially for migratory species that have a limited season in which to rear young able to join in the fall southern migration. In long-lived birds especially, this effort can be best organized if the parents work together efficiently. If pairs of a migratory species are bonded, they can breed earlier in the season because they do not have to hunt for and court a partner; their young have more time to grow strong before they must fly south. A seasoned pair has learned how to raise their young effectively; for example, who will take which shift in incubating the eggs and then in foraging for food for the nestlings: "Each pair must work out its own rhythm, which takes some time to perfect and gives the advantage to established couples" (Burger, 2001). Bonded couples are far more likely to raise young successfully than are non-bonded pairs.

In social mammals when male and female young are born into the same litter, they tend to bond together as they grow up, constantly in each other's presence. When they reach puberty, however, members of one sex or the other usually disperse from their natal group; this breaking of the brother–sister bond prevents inbreeding. In human beings, there is no such dispersal. An inborn incest taboo prevents a brother and sister from mating, but often the two remain close friends throughout their lives, which are enriched by this relationship.

This chapter will discuss bonding first in six primates (baboons, Japanese monkeys, bonobos gorillas, gibbons, and brown lemurs) who have evolved various types of intimacy among their members, and then in two birds, geese and petrels. These friendships all continue or occur outside of periods when copulation takes place, and so are disconnected from physical sex.

OLIVE AND CHACMA BABOONS

Barbara Smuts was a pioneer in elevating the importance of friendship in animals when she published her book *Sex and Friendship in Baboons* in 1985. Smuts, who trained at Stanford University in California, had a traumatic start to her career as an animal behaviorist (Ghiglieri, 1988). In 1975 when based at Jane Goodall's chimpanzee camp at Gombe, she and three other researchers were kidnapped by 40 guerrillas of the Marxist Popular Revolutionary Party from Zaire who had motored across Lake Tanganyika at midnight, hoping to capture Goodall herself. Smuts was chosen to carry ransom demands to the Tanzania government and Stanford University, which eventually resulted in ransom being paid and the other workers being freed. Rather than being soured on field research forever, Smuts turned her attention to the behavior of olive baboons (*Papio cynocephalus anubis*) living near Gilgil, Kenya.

Smuts (1985) describes Pandora and Virgil in the late afternoon, strolling along, slightly apart from the rest of the troop, stopping now and then to pick a handful of grass or dig up a bulb to chew. They are both in late middle age and members of the Eburru Cliffs baboon troop. Virgil, stuffed full of food, sits down to relax. Looking back, he sees Pandora and flashes the white patches of skin above his eyelids at her, the "come hither" look, at the same time alternately smacking his lips together and giving deep grunts. Pandora glances at him, returns the eye flashes, and hurries over to flop down on her back beside him. She dangles her leg in the air, presenting her flank so that Virgil will groom her. He does so carefully, parting the hairs on her belly and occasionally leaning forward to remove a bit of dead skin or dirt from her fur.

Then, becoming bored, he sinks to the ground and sighs. Pandora begins to groom him instead, working up his neck to his face, carefully removing bits of grit. Soon, Pandora's juvenile son, Plutarch, and infant daughter, Pyrrha, join the pair. Pyrrha amuses herself by jumping on Virgil's stomach as if he were a trampoline. At intervals, he opens his half-shut eyes, touching her gently with a finger to indicate he does not mind her exertions.

Night is coming, so at last Virgil rouses himself to clamber up the cliff face nearby, followed closely by Pandora and her family. Halfway up the cliff, he settles himself against a rock face, sitting upright, holding his toes in his hands and sinking his head onto his chest. He is ready to sleep. Pandora sits down beside him, her hand on his knee and her head against his shoulder. The two youngsters squeeze in between them. They will stay this way all night. Pandora and Virgil have been fast friends for at least five years, feeding together in the daytime and sleeping together at night; their closeness has little to do with sex, because most of the time she is either pregnant or lactating, and therefore not interested in mating.

Special friendships are not restricted to older baboons such as Pandora and Virgil. Nearby on the cliffs are two adolescents, Thalia and Alexander, sitting about five meters (16 ft) apart. Thalia was born in the troop but Alexander had transferred into it only a few months earlier. Alexander is facing west as if watching the setting sun. Thalia is nervously grooming herself, peeking over at Alexander every few seconds without turning her head. She grooms less and less as she turns her attention to him. When Alexander glances at her, she examines her foot; when he looks away, she gazes at him again. At last, without looking at her, Alexander begins to edge toward her. When he finally catches her eye, he gives her the "come hither" signal and grunts. Thalia freezes, then stares directly at him. As he comes closer, she turns to present her rump to him, peering nervously back over her shoulder. He grasps her hips, making loud lip-smacking noises, and then presents his side for grooming. She sets to work, gradually becoming calmer. They are still together the next morning when Smuts returns to the troop. This encounter marked not only the beginning of a close friendship between the two young baboons, but also the first sign of integration of Alexander into his new troop because of it.

Studies by hundreds of zoologists have shown that such male–female friendships are, in fact, a central feature of savannah baboon societies. In eight studies published before Smuts wrote her book, special friends are referred to variously as "godfathers,"

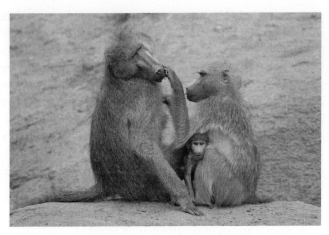

Figure 1. A female grooming a male chacma baboon.
© photolibrary.com

"associates," "constant associates," "friendships," "special relationships," "pair-bonds," "persistent high-frequency bonds," and "conspicuous dyadic relationships" (Smuts, 1985). Before this time, studies of the behavior of social mammals had concentrated largely on competition between males for the chance to mate with females in estrus, and reproductive behavior between males and receptive females.

Shirley Strum (1987) notes that, in 1973, when she described the baboon friendships she had observed between male and female dyads, often along with infants, and the fact that the males did not have a meaningful dominance hierarchy, other zoologists treated her observations with disdain. It was widely believed at that time that baboon males did have a dominance hierarchy; it made sense because the alpha males, as the most successful individuals, would pass their virile genes to the next generation by doing most of the mating. But the theory did not impress Smuts, who knew that low-ranking baboons also mated. There were other questions, though. Why did so many males spend so much time with females who were not sexually receptive? Why did the males play with and become close buddies with the youngsters of these females?

In theory, there are various reasons why a male baboon (and probably other primate males living in large multimale and female groups) would be buddies with one or more females (Smuts, 1985):

- This would help him integrate into a new troop after he left his natal one.
- He probably increases his mating opportunities.
- He becomes acquainted with an infant that could be his, and is able to protect it.
- He can use a female or infant held to his chest as a buffer to deter attack from another male.
- He makes allies among the females.

After many, many months of observations and note-taking on the daily activities of the members of the Eburru Cliffs troop, Smuts came to a number of conclusions – she had defined Friends (with a capital F) as those male–female couples who spent large amounts of time in grooming activity and in proximity to each other:

- All but one of the females had one or several male Friends, and most males, especially those who had been in the troop for a long time, had from one to six female Friends.
- Friend pairs belonged to more or less the same age group.
- Females groomed their male Friends more than the males groomed them, and therefore put more energy into maintaining the relationship.
- Females liked to be near their Friends and did not hesitate to approach and stay with them.
- Of all possible pair-bonds between males and anestrus females (either pregnant or lactating, but not sexually receptive) in the troop, only 12 percent represented Friendships.
- Male Friends became very attached to the females' offspring, greeting, holding, carrying, and grooming them.
- Females, who avoided non-Friend males, expressed fear, submission, or appeasement behavior if such a male came too close.
- Females had a reason to fear male baboons in general. On average, each put up with five male aggressive episodes a week, usually threats and chases, but one-quarter of them physical attacks. Each had, on average, one serious wound every year, defined as "a cut at least 3 cm long and deep enough to cause a gaping, bloody gash." These episodes could only be observed during the daytime and therefore were a minimum that took place; others may have occurred at night.
- Although a female and her young were often protected by her Friend from aggression by other males or females, the female

could not always count on him to be friendly. Sometimes he used her or especially her infant as a shield or buffer, knowing that a rival male would not hurt an infant. Sometimes another male harassed her because of a grievance with her male Friend.

Perhaps the most touching observations were those of male Friends cuddling, playing with or baby-sitting the infants of their female Friends. Strum describes the old male, Sumner, Friend of both long-term buddies, Peggy and Constance. He was an impressive animal with thick fur and large canines, but he was gentleness itself with a youngster: "Infants flocked around him and females relaxed when he was near." Pebbles, Peggy's infant, liked to play on Sumner. She would burrow through his thick fur, climb up his legs, and slide down his big belly. She would clamber over his face, struggling to reach the back of his neck while straddling his muzzle. As she grew older, she made flying leaps onto or off Sumner, using him as a springboard. Whenever he was playing with one of Peggy's or Constance's youngsters, other female baboons who wanted to be involved too, first asked permission from him as they would have from Peggy – "a glance, a present, and a lipsmack to the 'guardian,' then, unless told otherwise, a grunt, glance and touch to the infant." How wonderful to see a photograph of a huge, fierce male nuzzling the stomach of a tiny infant while its mother looks calmly on (Smuts, 1985). If these infants later, as juveniles, became orphaned by the death of their mother, the erstwhile male Friend would often take over the role as their primary adult companion (Cheney and Seyfarth, 2007).

Behaviors only persist in a group if they have evolutionary value. Smuts concluded that Friendships in baboons benefited both males and females, with their relationship being a type of social reciprocity. The females gained most because males are larger and more aggressive, and therefore a most useful long-term ally, who would usually prevent attacks on a female and her young by both females and males; each infant, after all, represents an enormous output of time and energy on the part of its mother. Females also had a chum with whom to hang out and share activities, as Pandora and Virgil exemplified.

Resident males benefited by Friendships, too. They were more likely than other males to mate with their Friend when she came into estrus and, therefore, father her youngsters. They could use her and her infants as a buffer to fend off attacks by other males. Additionally, because they were close to these infants and cared for them, they may have benefited their own progeny (although it is improbable that they could know this). For males newly transferring into the troop, females who might become their Friends, as we have seen for Thalia and Alexander, were important in helping integrate them into their new community. Shirley Strum (1987) notes that transferring males lacked both social ties and experience in their new troop. What they did have was aggression, which made them feared and unattractive to females. Short-term male residents were learning the ropes about how to get along within the troop, while long-term, older residents were the most successful with the females, although low ranked and least aggressive.

Sherlock is an example of social strategy that worked well in soliciting interest from a possible female Friend. He was an old baboon who had had plenty of time to perfect his strategy (Smuts, 2000). When sitting near an unattached female, if she suddenly glanced toward him twice in a row, he would start to concentrate on eating leaves. If she leaned a little bit away from him, he would take a step back, glancing about nonchalantly. If she caught his eye and did not look away, he would grunt softly and flash a mild "come-hither" flick of his eyelids, but otherwise remain where he was. He would approach and touch her only if she made a "come-hither" flash back at him. She would be friendly toward him and, in time, would willingly mate with him. Smuts summarizes his method, which might easily work with other species such as ourselves, as to "carefully observe the other, express your friendly intentions, keep your overtures subtle, and wait for the fearful one to make the first move."

Ryne Palombit and colleagues (1997) found that free-ranging chacma baboons (*Papio cynocephalus ursinus*) in southern Africa had similar male–female Friendships as did their relatives in East Africa, with whom Barbara Smuts and Shirley Strum were well acquainted. In this group, however, the need to combat infanticide seemed greater. Almost all lactating mothers of young infants formed strong bonds with one or two males with whom they had copulated before becoming pregnant, but if their infant died, the females ended this pair-bond. The researchers carried out several experiments that highlighted this facet of the Friendship bond:

(a)   In one test, they played auditory screams of the female Friends, to which the male Friends reacted more strongly than did other males.

(b)   Males also responded more strongly to the screams of their Friends than to the screams of other females.

(c)   Following an infant's death, however, the male Friend responded less strongly than did other males to their female Friend's screams.

(d)   Finally, male Friends responded more strongly than control males to playback sequences in which the female Friend's screams were combined with threat calls of a potentially infanticidal alpha male, but not when her screams were combined with threat calls of a non-infanticidal male or the alpha female.

The researchers conclude that the benefits of Friendships for females in this baboon troop derived from the need to protect their young against infanticide. Lactating females who were able to establish a close Friendship with a male suffered less stress as a result, with significantly lower glucocorticoid levels (Cheney and Seyfarth, 2007).

This same group of researchers published further research results on the chacma baboons in 2001. Sometimes two females competed for the attention of one male Friend. If one were dominant, even if she were much younger, she claimed greater proximity and grooming activity from the Friend than did the other female who was left, in large part, out in the cold. Because of this setback, the subordinate female made two compensatory changes in her life. First, she reduced any contact she had with a potentially infanticidal alpha male. Second, especially if she were fairly old, she not only cut back her association and grooming time with her male Friend, but she also spent more time associating with her maternal relatives. Presumably, these relatives would support her against any attack on her infant.

JAPANESE MONKEYS AND PECULIAR-PROXIMATE RELATIONS

Japanese monkeys (*Macaca fuscata*) have been a favorite subject of scientists interested in animal behavior. They were first studied in Japan after the Second World War when sweet potatoes were spread on open ground near forests to lure the monkeys out to where they could be observed. With feeding, the number of animals grew so large that they became a pest for nearby homes and farms. Rather than shoot them, a large number were shipped from the Arashiyama East area of Japan to a large ranch in Texas, forming a second research community called Arashiyama West (Fedigan, 1991). Today, important research continues with both East and West troops.

Yukio Takahata (1982) spent nearly three years watching the behavior of adults in the Arashiyama B Japanese monkey troop in Japan, especially noting which animals spent time resting and grooming together. Near the start of the project in April 1976, the troop had 210 adult members of whom eight were males over ten years of age and 84 females at least four and a half years old. The animals were fed five times a day with a handful of wheat and maize thrown on the ground about every 1.5 meters (5 ft). At each clump, a male and a female or a mother and her offspring often fed together.

Troops of Japanese monkeys may be very large, but the number of social encounters between individuals was few. Most females and males kept apart from each other unless the female was in estrus or monkeys were crowding around feeding stations, with one type of exception. Peculiar-proximate relations (PPRs) between male and female dyads was the third most common type of friendship, after the most common mother–daughter relationships and sibling friendships, especially by young monkeys. A PPR, which was present in about ten percent of all possible adult male–female dyads, is defined as a male–female relationship in which the pair were much more likely than other dyads to be close together and/or grooming each other. This would seem, on the surface, to be similar to the special Friend category for olive baboons discussed previously. However, a startling difference is that even though PPR dyads were almost always unrelated, they virtually never copulated, which seems odd from an evolutionary standpoint. Indeed, the pair did not usually hang out together at all when she was in estrus. But why should not males and females be friends without sex being involved?

A PPR offers several benefits to the female beyond that of simple companionship. Having a PPR gives a low-ranking female status. When she is physically near her partner, she can dominate a high-ranking female and so obtain more food. This has been called the "proximity effect." Additionally, her male can help her win battles. If a male intervenes between his PPR female and a non-PPR female who are squabbling, he is much more likely to side with his female no matter who is at fault. One male may have several related females as PPRs who, when they are crowded around him, may themselves seem to be friends.

However, in one case when a male died, his female PPRs quickly went their separate ways. (Many females do have special friendships with other females though, as described in the chapter: *In sisterhood*.)

In general, females seemed more keen than males to be in a PPR. For example, females groomed their PPR males more often than the males groomed them, although the males sometimes groomed infants. For another, if after they were together for a while the male partner moved away, the female often followed him, but the reverse was not true as the male seldom followed her. (Of course, a male could have many PPRs and would not be able to follow all of them, especially if he were high ranking.) However, the highly popular Male-59 frequently hung out with Momo, an ancient and senile female who finally died at about the age of 27 years. Like other PPRs, he was not related to her, but he often groomed her.

BONOBOS

Bonobos (*Pan paniscus*), originally called pygmy chimpanzees, were officially declared a distinct species in 1933, although they had been known by Europeans much earlier. The problem was that they so resembled the more common chimpanzees living in East Africa, *Pan troglodytes*, that the two apes were thought to be subspecies sharing, as they did (along with human beings), over 98 percent of DNA sequences (Furuichi and Thompson, 2008). Bonobos were originally famous for their paired female dalliances, but recent research from Lomako, Democratic Republic of Congo shows that male–female pairs may be even closer friends than female duos, with their bonds lasting on average longer than those of female pairs (Hohmann *et al.*, 1999). This was true for both related or unrelated protagonists. The males benefited by close bonds because of more sex and the sharing of the female's higher rank (females are dominant in this species) while the females benefited from copulations, reduced food competition, and protection against male harassment.

G. Hohmann and his colleagues (1999) gathered data from members of the Eyengo community, Lomako, which comprised about 12 males and 22 females, all of them recognizable by distinctive coloring or disfigured limbs. Their genetic relationships were largely known through analysis of mitochondrial and nuclear DNA extracted from fecal samples from each animal. Observations, carried out for about six months over four consecutive years, centered on grooming relationships of dyads and on 255 days of records of animal groups that showed what pairs of individuals tended to be present together. During each field season there were more male–female pairs (over 50%) than (shorter-lasting) female–female pairs (25%–41%) and few male duos. Close pairs groomed each other more often than random pairs, reciprocated more within the grooming, and groomed for longer. Data from bonobos at the site of Wamba, Zaire, also show strong male–female bonds. Perhaps the male–female bonds present in earlier studies of bonobo communities were overlooked because of the astonishing joyousness of the sexual behavior among the females.

MOUNTAIN GORILLA

As is widely known, Dian Fossey, backed by the anthropologist and paleontologist L.S.B. Leakey, was the second person after Jane Goodall to dedicate her life to observing her favorite animal, in her case mountain gorillas (*Gorilla gorilla beringei*) in the Virunga Mountains of Rwanda. She arrived in 1967, set up camp, and stayed until she was murdered there in 1985 (Mowat, 1987). Gorillas are closely related to chimpanzees but their social life is different, presumably because they eat common herbage that is readily available in massive amounts. A group of about ten can always find enough food for the day within a few hectares, so there is little ecological pressure operating against group cohesion (Ghiglieri, 1988). Gorilla families live mainly in one-male troops where the female adults may develop lifelong bonds with the male. Such was the case with Effie, the alpha female of group 5 (Fossey, 1983). In 1969 Beethoven, a 160 kg (350 lb) silverback, was the alpha male with four adult females in his troop who mated exclusively with him. Fossey did not know how they had all come together because she had only recently met them. The troop included Idano, Liza, Marchessa, and their young, but Effie was Beethoven's favorite. Together they raised five healthy youngsters thanks to her "patience, stability, strong maternal instincts, and outstanding closeness with Beethoven." Effie's children, along with Effie, always stayed near him where he could watch the youngsters playing. Over the years, the other females left the troop: Idano suffered a fatal infection in 1973, Liza emigrated four years later because Beethoven would not mate with her, and Marchessa died of ill-health in 1980. But Effie lived on. In contrast to hamadryas baboon couples where the female is forced by the male to remain with him, Effie was happy to stay with Beethoven because, as far as Fossey could tell, she loved him.

Effie had a strong personality and, as an alpha female willing to fight, usually got what she wanted for herself and her young (Weber and Vedder, 2001). She had priority when obtaining clay and roots to eat, and even Beethoven sometimes yielded to her when she wanted to follow a different trail than the others, or find a better nesting site. But not always, as Amy Vedder, one of Fossey's research students, noticed one day while she was carrying out research for her doctorate, which involved recording what plants gorillas were eating for five or six hours each day. (By the end of her study, she had logged 2000 hours in this activity!) When Beethoven happened to look over and see Effie helping herself to the fruit at a juicy blackberry bush, he immediately cough-grunted and rushed over to demand the fruit for himself, in the process pushing Vedder aside and injuring her leg. He may even have bitten Effie, who quickly fled the scene.

On two documented occasions, however, Effie refused to give Beethoven what he wanted, which was to get out of the rain. Once, a sudden storm caught group 5 unprepared. As the rain pelted down, Effie, followed by two younger gorillas, crowded under a huge *Hagenia* log along with two researchers, Bill Weber and Amy Vedder (2001). Beethoven was left in the rain for a few minutes before striding over to the others hoping to squeeze in with them. He stood in front of Effie, pursing his lips, but she did not react. Instead, she sat tight, finally giving a dismissive series of sharp cough-grunts. Beethoven did not respond for a minute or two, but then went elsewhere to find shelter. (The two humans wondered what on earth they would have done had Effie not refused Beethoven's mute request.) Another time, after he had built himself a sloppy day nest that did not keep out the rain, he tried to move into Effie's protected nest where she and two of her offspring were happily dozing (Fossey, 1983). Effie refused to move over and give him room in the crowded quarters at first, but later she let him squeeze in behind her, although where much of his body remained hanging over the nest edge.

Effie and Beethoven lived to a ripe old age, dying finally of natural causes. Beethoven had sired at least 19 young, and Effie was survived by at least seven offspring and two great grandchildren. Theirs was a comfortable and steadfast friendship that lasted at least 15 years.

GIBBONS

Gibbons, comprising at least twelve species in the family Hylobatidae, are small apes from south-east Asia who have a social organization rare, if not unique, among primates (Bartlett, 2007). They live in three-dimensional defended territories large enough to encompass sufficient fruit-bearing trees to provide their food. Until recently, gibbons were described as monogamous, as couples were commonly seen raising young together in a family group. This was thought to be a commendable arrangement because of its similarity with human families. However, close study indicates this is a simplification. In general, both males and females may seek sex from mates beyond their border, sometimes their young play with young from neighboring territories, and the family is not necessarily a nuclear one as was believed (Bartlett, 2009). Instead, it can better be called a household unit that may include non-related adult animals.

A comparison of the pair activity of the white-handed gibbons (*Hylobates lar*) and of the larger siamangs (*Hylobates syndactylus*) by Ryne Palombit (1996) gives an idea of species' variation. Siamangs had more instances of close proximity between pairs, more relaxed physical contact, more embracing, and more communal use of sleep trees. They also groomed each other fairly equitably, undoubtedly strengthening their pair-bond in this way. For the gibbon pairs, the males did most of the grooming while the females tended to ignore male requests to be groomed in turn. Palombit indicates that male guarding may have been the selection force behind the original pair-bonds in both species.

What about special friendships? Gibbons are difficult to observe in the wild because they are small (about 5 or 6 kg, 11 to 13 lb), high above the ground, and very agile, swinging from branch to branch by virtue of their extremely long arms and mobile shoulder joints. Even if you can see them, you cannot see many of their interactions. We do know that pairs are often near each other, jointly defend their territory, and practice mutual grooming. However, in one study lar gibbon males spent more time grooming young gibbons than they did grooming adult females (Bartlett, 2009), and partner changes were so frequent that monogamous pairings were serial at best. Volker Sommer and Ulrich Reichard (2000) believe that a monogamous pair of gibbons living together for their whole lives is perhaps a non-existent concept. For this reason, gibbon relationships are also considered briefly in the chapter: *Family and group tight bonds*, which discusses group friendships.

Duetting, performed by heterosexual duos of at least ten and probably by all gibbon species, is "an interactively organized pair display in which one pair partner coordinates its vocalizations in time with those of the other" (Méndez-Cárdenas and Zimmermann, 2009). Over 200 species of birds and some monogamous monkeys and lemurs as well as gibbons sing, call, or shout out their duets.

We know most about the actual duetting process itself from the behavior of siamang gibbons living in captivity. Observers at the

Louisiana Purchase Gardens and Zoo in the United States were amazed when their eighteen-year-old male was immediately turned on by a six-year-old female newly added to the zoo (Maples *et al.*, 1989). He had been captured in the wild as an infant, lived as a couple for five years before his partner died, then spent the past twelve years alone. Siamang couples announce their pairship by singing loud and elaborate duets described as follows (McCarthy, 2004):

> The male gives two deep booms, the female then booms once, the male booms twice again, "and the female must immediately come in with accelerating high-frequency barks. After about the fifth bark, the male should utter an ascending boom, the female's barks should speed up, and the male should do a bitonal scream. At once the female must start another series of barks, and after five the male should do a scream, this time a ululating scream. The female does some fast high barks, then both of them bark and hurtle about."

The Louisiana Zoo pair began to practice this duet right away as a testament to their friendship, their performance improving quickly. Over a three-month period, the percentage of started great-call sequences that were correctly completed rose from 24% to 79%, and finally almost all were perfect. "One of the most common mistakes was for the female to start her first set of accelerating high barks without waiting for the male's second double boom. The other common mistake was for the male to bungle his bitonal scream, giving either the ululating scream or the locomotion call instead." (McCarthy, 2004.)

Perhaps duetting initially enables each partner to assess the behavior and vigor of the other as a suitable mate. Maybe it serves to alert each to where the other is in dense vegetation and helps coordinate their activities. Possibly, it warns other animals of the same species that a territory is occupied by two individuals who will defend it. Certainly, it is a euphoric display of togetherness.

RUFOUS LEMUR

Three essentials for any successful species are safety, food, and reproduction. Without the first two, an animal will not survive, and without the third, neither will the species. Female ring-tailed lemurs (as well as most other lemurs) gain these necessities by being dominant to males, as we shall see in the chapter: *Mothers and daughters*; their dominance ensures that they and their offspring usurp the best forage available and are safe from male aggression. It is the female who chooses with whom she will mate.

Rufous or red-fronted lemurs (*Eulemur fulvus rufus*), although they are fairly closely related to ring-tailed lemurs (and for a long time were believed to belong to the same genus), have adopted a fundamentally different reproductive strategy, that of females sharing equality with males rather than being dominant to them. Rufous females are much less strongly attached to their female kin than are ringtails. Instead, they often team up with a male, forming "special relationships," the term used in a scientific paper on the topic by Michael Pereira and Catherine McGlynn (1997). For their research, the authors observed the social behavior, over seven months, of two partly overlapping troops of these lemurs living in a very large forested enclosure at the Duke University Primate Center in the United States. All the lemurs were well habituated to human voyeurs and had either colored collars, pendants, or distinctive features so that each was known individually.

The authors circulated on foot among the troop every few days, keeping at least three meters (10 ft) away from any animal and making notes on a check sheet of four types of behavior for each of their focal individuals: (a) approaches when a lemur moved to within 2.5 meters (8 ft) of a non-moving lemur, (b) departures when a lemur moved away from within a 2.5 meter distance from the other, (c) grooming when a lemur made repeated strokes over another's pelage using its dental comb and/or tongue, and (d) agonistic interactions whenever a focal animal exchanged either aggressive or submissive behavior with a troop-mate. If a third party mixed into a social conflict, this was recorded too, as was the nearness of other group members to the focal subject, at five minute intervals. At the end of the study, they had between seven and eight hours of focal sampling for each adult. Each of the four adult females was especially friendly with one unrelated or distantly related adult male, staying close with mutual grooming (which could be traded for other favors [Port *et al.*, 2009]), and fairly often supporting him with only the occasional squabble.

While the better-known ring-tailed lemur advertises her period of estrus with a swollen vulva, the rufous female's ovulation period is concealed, as it also is in women. The rufous female certainly mates with her long-time friend, but perhaps with a few other males as well. The researchers report that together the duo forms a team: she backs him in aggressive interactions with other lemurs and he backs her, although eventually a female may choose a replacement special friend if the male becomes unsupportive of her or too old for her tastes. They note that such dyads obviate the need for females to be dominant, as is the case in most lemur species, and conclude that "the male–female pair is the fundamental social unit of *Eulemur fulvus*."

But wait a minute. This is not the final word. Deborah Overdorff reports a year later (1998) that the male–female relationships could better be described as "dyads" rather than anything more intense. For 17 months, she had observed rufous lemur behavior in two wild groups in Madagascar. With a view to testing possible pair-bonds between the sexes, she consulted her data, asking and answering four questions:

(a)   Were pair-bonds stable throughout the year? No, she found they were not.

(b)   Were the bonds enhanced during the mating season (to ensure the female mated only with her buddy) and during the birth season (when her infant might be in danger of infanticide)? No, they were not.

(c)   Did the female mate exclusively or more often with her special friend than with other males? No, she did not.

(d)   Were rates of aggression highest during the mating and birth seasons, as the special friend combats other males who want to mate with his female and when there is a possibility of infanticide – the Infanticide Prevention Hypothesis?

Fights did increase in the groups during the mating season, some owing to general tension but some because a special male did try to keep other males away from his partner. No lemur tried to attack an infant though, so the infanticide hypothesis was not supported. Indeed, infanticidal attempts have not been observed in this species. We can conclude that male and female rufous lemurs tend to form close friendship pairs, but these are not as tight as had been presumed.

GEESE

It is heartening in our monogamous society to think that geese mate for life, and usually this is true, as Konrad Lorenz relates in his book *Here I am – Where Are You? The Behavior of the Greylag Goose* (1991). When he was a little boy, Lorenz at first wanted to be an owl, because owls could stay up all night. But from his bedtime reading about wild geese, it occurred to him that owls could neither swim nor dive, which he had recently learned to do, so he decided that he would be an aquatic bird instead. When he realized that he could not actually *become* such a bird, he determined instead to own one, so his family gave him a baby duckling to raise. His interest in the development of this little charge would lead him to research, in exquisite detail, the behavior of greylag geese. His findings would win him a Nobel Prize in 1973.

Lorenz's observations made after his retirement in 1973 focus in part on the fast friendship of Mercedes and Florian, a pair of greylag geese (*Anser anser*) living on a pond near Grünau and Lake Alm in Austria. Mercedes hatched at the beginning of May 1979 and was raised, along with three siblings, by her biological parents. At the age of one year, she separated from her parents and, by the spring of 1982, was more or less a free agent. Enter Florian, who had hatched in 1973 and been unlucky in love, in friendship, and in combat over the next nine years. In February 1982, Florian bested Mercedes' suitor Nilson in an exhausting, violent duel with their wing shoulders, then ran to Mercedes while uttering as loud a triumph call as he could muster, given his recent strenuous battle; Mercedes responded positively to him thus cementing their pair-bond. The triumph call is usually given after a male swims or runs aggressively with his neck stretched forward toward a rival, who turns and flees. The victor then rushes back to the female who has been the cause of the dispute, wings outstretched as human arms would be after a soccer goal, at which they both utter loud triumph calls with their heads very close together and near the ground. These are followed by rolling calls and soft cackling sounds made by both geese. Lorenz notes that "The motivational force that drives each of these birds to perform the triumph ceremony with its partner appears to be overwhelming."

From this time on, Mercedes and Florian were a bonded pair. They did not have young in their first spring together, but in 1983 they hatched six goslings from six eggs, leading their offspring from the nest site to a lake seven kilometers (4 mi) away where all six successfully fledged. The next year they raised five young, the members of the family so closely attuned that they could be recognized at a distance when in flight. In 1985, Lorenz reduced the clutch incubated to four eggs, from which three young survived. At the beginning of 1986, these three and their parents were still a closely knit family; but Florian and Mercedes did not breed that year and one of their youngsters from 1985 joined the group. The parents remained bonded at least until 1987, when Lorenz was writing his book, which would be published in German the following year.

Most geese mate for life, but many of these romances do not last very long, as Lorenz found among his large flocks of greylag geese. Many females died prematurely, especially during the incubation season, from natural predators or disease, to which they were susceptible because of the stress of reproduction. This meant that about half of all paired males lost their mate during their lifetime. By contrast, only about 20 percent of females lost their partner. For the 32 ganders whose mate was gone, more than half formed pair-bonds with a new female. Somewhat less than a third remained alone initially, while the rest formed fast friendships with other males. Of the females who lost their mate, three-quarters of them formed a new pair-bond, with only a quarter remaining alone.

Not all pair-bonds were sacrosanct. Occasionally, geese changed partners. Out of 61 females, as many as 15 left their first mate to form a pair-bond with another gander in the following season. There seemed to be good reason for this: for nine of these females this happened after a failed attempt at breeding, and in four other cases the pairs did not breed at all. In only two cases did geese change partners after having successfully raised young.

Bernd Heinrich (2004) describes the vicissitudes of partner change as it affected Pop, Peep, and acquaintances, Canada geese (*Branta canadensis*) who nested on a bog in Vermont where he kept close watch over them for several years. Peep was hatched in 1998 from an egg of a wild Canada goose put under a domestic goose to incubate. She grew up in a farmyard, a chaotic surrounding for her, her name commemorating the loud insistent noises she made when she was separated from humans upon whom she was partly imprinted. By fall, she was full grown and wild enough to join a migrating flock of geese heading south. To Heinrich's delight, she returned to his bog the following second spring, accompanied by a male whom he called Pop. That year, 2000, Peep and Pop nested and produced four eggs, none of which hatched following a major battle with another pair of geese on the bog.

During the 2001 spring migration, geese returned to Vermont, but this time Pop had a new mate, Jane, who had nested in the same bog the year before with another male. Perhaps all geese are not faithful to their mate, Heinrich thought. Or had Peep acted out of goose-character because she had been partly imprinted on human beings in her infancy? Yet it was Pop who seemed to be the unfaithful one. When he and Jane had been back in Vermont a week, Peep flew in to be greeted by Pop, but she was attacked time after time by a jealous Jane. Pop seemed conflicted at first, paying attention to Peep when Jane was away by joining her in a bathing routine in which they jointly splashed about in the water. But when Jane flew back, he again teamed up with her. Pop chose Jane, but he could not bring himself to chase Peep away. Jane, by contrast, did everything in her power to evict Peep from the area, which she succeeded in doing as she was far more aggressive than her rival. Heinrich believes that if Pop and Peep had arrived back at their bog, their home of the previous year, at the same time, they might have still been a couple. It seems timing can be crucial.

In mid-April, a gander who seemed to be Jane's former partner, Jack, flew to the bog. (Heinrich had not banded the geese or given them distinctive markings, so he had to tell them apart by their small physical differences and by their behavior.) Pop attacked Jack ferociously, chasing him away from Jane. Jack was joined in flight by Peep! Then Pop and Jane together chased away the two rivals. Heinrich believed that Peep and Jack had perhaps bonded and flown elsewhere to nest, while Pop and Jane remained as the only breeding geese on his bog that summer, along with their five healthy goslings. Strangely, one summer day Heinrich saw them not with five goslings but with ten! Another pair of geese must have walked to the pond with their family (the goslings were too young to fly) and then flown away from all parental duties.

Fortunately, parenting is not high-intensity for geese and other large waterfowl. Their young are able to look after themselves on hatching, immediately hunting on their own for grass and aquatic plants to eat. The role of the gander (and the female to a lesser extent) is not to bring food back to the nest, but to protect the new fledglings from rival geese, hawks, eagles, skunks, raccoons, and foxes. Heinrich saw ganders attack and chase away various dogs and a fox that threatened their young. For swans and cranes as well as geese, all of whom are large adults with precocial young, it is imperative that a male stay with them to keep them safe so they can grow to adulthood and carry on his genetic heritage. For large waterfowl that breed in northern countries, there is no possibility of having a second mating in the short summer season, and reproduction begins early. For smaller birds that produce precocial young such as ducks, quail, grouse, rails, and many sandpipers who can hide easily because of their small size, the males leave their mates after the female has laid her eggs. They would not be able to combat predators even if they were present. If there is a chance of having a second set of young during the summer, the males are free to be involved in that, too.

In his book *The Swans* (1972), Peter Scott, son of the Antarctic explorer, notes that for the largely non-migratory mute swans (*Cygnus olor*) in central England, few change partners while their mate is still alive. The low rate of "divorce" was three percent for pairs that had already bred and nine percent for pairs that had not yet bred or had failed to breed. For northern Bewick's swans (*Cygnus columbianus bewickii*), the pair-bond is even stronger. This species does migrate, so that time is of the essence in preparing a nest, laying and incubating eggs, and raising strong young ready to fly south in the fall. Scott notes that all these activities must be "closely synchronised, rapidly initiated and intensely performed." Pairs that stay together will provide the best parental care and be most productive, even though their earlier attempts at breeding may not have been successful. There is said to be no divorce among members of this species (Masson, 1999).

William Henry Hudson (1923), who lived for many years in Argentina, relates a story told to him by a sheep farmer there. This man had seen in August, early spring, two geese (species unspecified), one walking south and the other sometimes walking and sometimes flying back and forth, screaming in excitement. The former turned out to be a female who had broken her wing and could not fly. The frantic escort was her partner who desperately wanted her to migrate with him south to the Magellanic Islands where they could start their family. Despite his anguish, he would not leave her and fly on alone. This is a tale that was bound to end badly, but it depicts the close bond that can exist between a pair of mated geese.

GREY-FACED PETREL

Grey-faced petrel couples (*Pterodroma macroptera gouldi*), like many penguin pairs, spend most of their time apart, despite their necessarily close bond. These handsome, dark-colored birds with a meter-wide (3 ft) wingspan breed mainly on the volcanic Whale Island off the north east coast of New Zealand. Researcher Mike Imber (1976) of the New Zealand Wildlife Service found, by catching and banding birds, that during courtship a male takes possession of a burrow about March, where his mate of the previous year will soon join him for a few days of quality time. They copulate, then fly (presumably separately, given the presence of winds and dark nights) over 600 km (375 mi) to the south east, well beyond the continental shelf where, judging from an analysis of stomach contents, they feed largely on cephalopods such as squids and other animals. Over 90 percent of their prey species are bioluminescent, coming to the surface of the ocean between dusk and dawn (Imber, 1973).

Two months later, the female returns to the same burrow to lay one huge egg weighing nearly one-fifth of her body weight. She incubates this egg for about four days before she is relieved by her mate. He sits on it for 17 days while she flies again to the far feeding grounds for food. She then replaces him for a second 17-day period when he feeds far away, after which he again replaces her. When she flies in after her 17-day forage, the cherished egg is about to hatch. There has been no time for the pair to relax together for this first phase of their parenthood, nor is there for the next 120 days during which they separately bring food for their chick about once a week. When the chick is finally able to fly away from the burrow it has called home, the pair has several months to unwind before they begin the whole child-rearing process all over again. Their behavior is obviously well synchronized to carry out their parental duties, but they do not have much time to savor their friendship.

As we have seen in this chapter, a variety of species have males and females who become long-term friends. The advantages of hetero-sexual friendship include companionship, allogrooming, joint parent-ing, patrolling territories together, support in aggressive encounters, prevention of infanticide, making an immigrating male feel at home, and a female gaining status from a dominant partner. Even so, such heterosexual bonding is not common in the animal kingdom.

Of all the species that have group and/or family structures, excluding therefore most amphibians, reptiles, fish, and invertebrates, it is almost always the females who care for their growing offspring, and it is also the females who are likely to form fast friendships with each other, as we shall see in the next chapter.

In sisterhood

What conditions foster close friendships between female duos? Certainly, they often flourish where adult females are familiar with each other. Sisters are often especially close (or might sibling rivalry sometimes carry on into adulthood, as it does in some women? Female infant spotted hyena siblings will fight until the death of the weaker if food is limited [Wahaj *et al.*, 2007]). The relationships of mothers and their adult daughters, who are often best buddies, will be considered in the chapter: *Mothers and daughters*.

Theoretically, social species develop bonds of friendship most strongly between same-sex partners in the sex that does not leave the group when it reaches puberty, thus avoiding the possibility of inbreeding. This makes sense. One would expect that individuals who have known each other for a lifetime will have the strongest potential for friendship. It applies to the much-researched olive baboons where males emigrate at puberty and the females stay in their natal troop, continuing friendships that have been in place since their infancy. It is also generally true for chimpanzees where males are more likely to be affiliated with other males than females with females; in this species as in gorillas, most (but not all) females transfer from their natal group into a new one during adolescence. At Gombe, Tanzania, once in their new troop as adults, female chimpanzees spent relatively little time together with the exception of the few special friends that interest us here (Goodall, 1986). But this theory is decidedly *not* true for bonobos. In this species, females emigrate at puberty, but when they join another group they form a remarkably strong gregarious sisterhood with their new female friends.

This chapter considers female friendships in six primates (bonobos, chimpanzees, gorillas, baboons, Japanese monkeys, and blue monkeys), two hoofed animals (horses and zebu), three carnivores (lions, hyenas, and grizzly bears), two cetaceans (dolphins and baleen whales), and one bird (Laysan albatross).

No females are more into each other than bonobos (*Pan paniscus*), and although they are closely related to chimpanzees, they inhabit different environments and behave in very different ways. Bonobos are much less well known than chimpanzees for several reasons: they are only found in the dense forests of the Congo River basin; they are much fewer in number; they do not fit in with the male-biased theory that "man" evolved to be hunters, power-oriented, and dominant to females; and one suggestion – that they were already near extinction so why should we bother about them? In reality, bonobos would seem to be more closely related than chimpanzees to humans: our body proportions are more similar, and bonobos and people share a propensity for friendly behavior that is absent in chimpanzees (de Waal, 2008).

When Takayoshi Kano (1992) from Japan began his studies of bonobos at Wamba, Zaire in 1973, their behavior was almost completely unknown, thanks in part to the dense vegetation there. Knowing that the future of the ape was bleak, given the rapidly increasing human population of Zaire, Kano made two important decisions. First, he decided to give the bonobos some food, sugar cane stalks, so that he could learn about them more quickly than if he had to habituate them to humans without any reward – a far longer process as the bonobo researchers at Lomako Forest in Zaire would discover. Second, no primatologist could come to work at Wamba without first learning the local language of the people there, Lingala (de Waal, 1997). The research team hired many local people who, in conversing with the scientists, came to be interested in the species and to care for the apes, rather than thinking of them as bush meat to be slaughtered for food. Sometimes in the evening, Kano and his colleagues would chat with villagers about what they were discovering about bonobos. There is a wonderful photograph in de Waal's book *Bonobos: The Forgotten Ape* (1997) of a large group of school children standing transfixed in a jungle, as three bonobos bound across the lane in front of them. This important policy of involving the local people continues, but bonobos are still at risk of extinction in various regions of Congo (Idani *et al.*, 2008).

A striking phenomenon about bonobo society is that females are dominant to males, even though the opposite is true for their close relative the chimpanzee (and most other mammals that have males larger than females). Amy Parish, an ardent bonobophile who earned her PhD from the University of California at Davis studying female bonding in captive bonobos (de Waal, 1997), has studied this in detail. She notes that female dominance upsets many people, especially men. If they see females bullying males in captivity, they try to stop it, even though males bullying females is seen as acceptable behavior in other species (*Bonobos: A Matriarchal Society*, 2006). Some scientists propose that males allowing themselves to be bullied by females means only that they are chivalrous. They call this behavior "strategic male deference" and postulate that the males do it to obtain more sex from the females (although sex from the females is freely given). Fast friends within bonobo communities include the rare category of mother–son duos (see the chapter: *Mothers and sons, and providing free food*).

When female bonobos move and settle into a new troop during adolescence, they too, like the older female residents, become dominant to males. Females, juveniles, and infants forage closely together, with rare squabbles. When they rest, the females often groom each other (which chimpanzee females do not do). They travel together too, along with males. At feeding sites, an adult female may forcefully steal sugar cane from another female, but neither needs to worry about aggression from the (inferior) males; and they often have sex, which will smooth over any friction. The only real wrestling matches between females occur when a female feels that she has to protect one of her sons (as we shall see in the chapter: *Mothers and sons, and providing free food*).

Some pairs of females form an especially close relationship sustained by sexual activity. One female eager for sex focuses on another by inviting her to have genito-genital contact (which is so common that researchers refer to it as "GG rubbing") (Kano, 1992). She does this by approaching her projected partner X casually, lingering a bit, and then sitting down beside her. Then she makes "a demand for invitation" by standing upright on two legs, extending her hand toward X, putting her face close to her friend's face, and peering into her eyes as if to say "Please join me in genital rubbing." Compliant X lies down on her back (the favored position for copulation with a male), and embraces the female with her arms when she climbs onto her stomach. Then, in this stomach-to-stomach position, they make quick, rhythmic, thrusting movements similar to those during copulation but more side-to-side, with their clitorises touching. Both their faces show "an uncontrollable emotion." The females end this activity with a sudden scream, similar to that emitted during copulation. Orgasms are surely an excellent cement for female friendships within the community. Indeed, Kano is convinced that the forward position of the genitals in female bonobos "evolved for GG rubbing rather than for ventral copulation." Bruce Bagemihl (1999) notes that "almost without exception, animals with 'different' sexualities and/or genders are completely integrated into the social fabric of their species, eliciting little of the attention, hostility, segregation, or secrecy that we are accustomed to associating with homosexuality in our society."

Gen'ichi Idani (1991) researched the specific topic of relationships between immigrant and resident female bonobos at Wamba, Zaire, because it is very often a young immigrant who transfers to a new troop just after her first period of estrus and focuses on a "specific senior female" (SSF) for individual attention. In chimpanzee troops, resident females act aggressively against new immigrant young females, but the opposite is true in bonobo groups. When the young immigrant has made contact with all the females in the troop, she chooses her SSF whom she approaches frequently, follows, and entices into grooming and GG rubbing activities. The SSF seems less keen than her young partner, but in reality, has more interaction with this new adolescent than with other resident females. Nao was fixated on Kame (mentioned in the chapter: *Mothers and sons, and providing free food*) until she had her first birth, but after that she no longer interacted much with her SSF. Idani concludes that the relationship of an immigrant with her SSF eases her integration into a troop. Female bonobos, unlike chimpanzees, tend to travel in stable groups, so it is important that they be familiar with and accepted by the other females as part of a stable community.

Females often have sex with males too, whether or not they are in estrus. Amy Parish decided to carry out an experiment at the San Diego Wild Animal Park with adult males, adult females, and young bonobos to see whether females preferred to be with males or other females (de Waal, 1997). The animals were put together in eight different groupings, with at least one male and two females always present. Interactions between individuals were then recorded. Parish found that females liked to be with females rather than males, sitting or playing together and grooming each other. Females followed a female around seven times more often than they followed a male. She was also able to observe bonobos fishing for honey at the Stuttgart Zoo. The female adults took feeding priority, but before they took advantage of the honey, they had sex among themselves:

"Sex apparently facilitated their relationship, thus helping them dominate the male."

Parish was amazed at the intelligence of bonobos when she began to collect fecal samples from them so that their hormonal composition could be analyzed (de Waal, 1997; *Bonobos: A Matriarchal Society*, 2006). She wanted to correlate the presence of estrogen and progesterone, which varies with their menstrual cycle, with the behavior of each female. When she saw the female Lana holding a turd, she held out her hand and wiggled her fingers as bonobos do when they are begging. At first, Lana did not know what Parish wanted, turning around and around and looking about her on the empty floor. Finally, she looked at the turd, noticed Parish staring at it, and held it out so that Parish could take it. Soon, without any reward, all four females were saving their fecal productions for her. Four years later, at the Stuttgart Zoo, a bonobo who had also been in the San Diego quarters as a youngster remembered that her mother had given Parish turds, even though she herself had not done so. She indicated this by presenting Parish with her own unusual gift, something she had never done before for anyone else. After a long absence, Parish again visited the San Diego Zoo with her small son Kalen, named after the first bonobo she had ever met. Lana was thrilled to see her old friend, standing erect, calling out, and clapping her hands. When she noticed Kalen at Parish's side, she became even more excited. She rushed over to pick up her own infant whom Parish had never seen, proudly holding him up suspended by his arms. She was showing Parish that not only had Parish had a child, but so had she. Parish is now closely connected with the Sankuru Nature Reserve in the Democratic Republic of Congo, a tropical rainforest larger in size than Belgium which is managed by indigenous people (*Bonobo Conservation Initiative*, 2006). Its mission is to preserve bonobos and okapis from extinction.

About every two hours, female bonobos participate in GG rubbing sessions lasting ten or fifteen seconds, so these activities are important socially. In her book *Evolution's Rainbow*, Joan Roughgarden (2004) summarizes ways in which they support female friendships:

- sex facilitates the sharing of food,
- sex facilitates reconciliation after a dispute,
- sex helps a young immigrant arrival integrate into her new group, and
- sex helps in the formation of coalitions to chase away harassing males or corral food.

By evolving a social behavior that enables females to control both access to food and the aggression of males, female bonobos begin to reproduce earlier in their lives than do female chimpanzees and therefore have, on average, a higher lifetime reproductive success.

Although bonobos and chimpanzees are closely related, their social systems are quite different. Chimpanzee females are reproductively receptive less than five percent of their adult lifetime, while for female bonobos it is close to 50 percent (de Waal, 1997). The menstrual cycle of a chimpanzee is about 35 days, while that of a bonobo is 45 days, during which the period of their genital swelling lasts much longer. In addition, unlike chimpanzees, bonobos resume sexual swelling within a year of giving birth, when they are sexually active but not fertile. During evolution, the use of sex in fostering social relationships between females has obviously become momentous in bonobos, but a non-starter for chimpanzees.

CHIMPANZEES[1]

Jane Goodall (1986) is celebrated for her pioneering research on the behavior of chimpanzees at Gombe, Tanzania. At first, in 1960, she worked alone, trailing animals through the forests; then she began giving them bananas so she could watch them more easily. From 1964 she was joined by a number of research assistants, and by 1975 there were 22 Tanzanian, European, and American students (both undergraduate and graduate) working with her. In that year, however, a group of rebels from Zaire kidnapped four members of the research team whom they held for ransom. They were eventually rescued, but from then the research was done mainly by Tanzanians as it was too dangerous for Europeans to be there. Goodall herself was restricted in the research she could carry out. However, her comprehensive book published in 1986 gives a wonderful record of all that had been discovered about her chimpanzees up to that time.

In social behavior, chimpanzees of Gombe are quite unlike bonobos despite their very similar DNA. Jane Goodall (1986) comments that the chimpanzees (*Pan troglodytes schweinfurthii*) she watched for many years had no unrelated special friends among the adult females. Chimpanzees have a fission–fusion society, in which members form groups that soon disband and reform again into different assemblages, and females at Gombe did not fraternize much with each other there.

However, she mentions a few friendships. For example, Circe and Nope were large females who may have been sisters. They played, groomed, hung out together, and supported each other in social conflicts. Circe became the alpha female after Goodall's favorite female Flo, but when Circe died in 1968, Nope did not take over the care of Circe's three-year-old daughter Cindy. With no one to look after her, Cindy died seven weeks later. Nope herself never made another close friend, but devoted herself to her family, nursing her second infant Lolita for seven years.

Flo and Olly, both older females (born about 1939 and 1929, respectively) also spent a good deal of time together, along with their families. Olly tended to be timid though, and when Figan and Faben, Flo's sons, began to challenge adult females, she started to avoid Flo and her sons. When mothers with juvenile young hang out together, each youngster benefits by having a friend to play with and by association with that friend's mother and her male friends (Williams *et al.*, 2002). This socialization suggests a substantial benefit for the youngster when she/he reaches adulthood and begins to interact with other adults.

When Goodall's definitive work on chimpanzees was published in 1986, it was generally assumed that a lack of friendships among female chimpanzees was the final word on this aspect of their social behavior. This agreed with reports from Japanese researchers at the nearby Mahale Mountains (Nishida, 1990). However, with further extensive research on this species in other parts of Africa, notably two areas much more forested than Gombe's more open woodland habitat and where the chimpanzees had not been provided with food by the researchers, we now know that there is much variation in possible female friendships (Boesch, 2002).

The first area is at Ngogo in the Kibale Forest of Uganda, where Michael Ghiglieri (1988) spent two years watching chimpanzees of the same race interact with each other while feeding in fruiting trees. These trees were huge; one mighty fig tree had 44 visits by chimpanzees in one day, the males and females usually arriving at different times. To the chimpanzees, such trees were much more than a large food patch – they were centers of fellowship, "almost catalysts of socialization for the apes." Presumably, the females became more friendly among themselves because they spent so much time together at these pleasant venues unknown at Gombe. Ghiglieri, who observed that Kibale females actually liked to be with each other and to groom together, gives seven reasons why this might be so:

(a)   Females were less dominant than males and so more fun to groom with – the more dominant an individual, the more likely they were to cheat in allogrooming, giving less grooming than they received.

(b)   Males, being bigger, managed to grab most of the food in short supply such as meat.

(c)   Females traveled less than did males who were often on boundary patrols, so they had more time to spend with their youngsters and friends.

(d)   Females were more likely than males to stay away from alien groups that might attack and endanger them and their young.

(e)   When females hung out together, their infants had an opportunity to play with each other, which improved their social skills.

(f)   A few females had kin ties, which bound them to members of their natal group.

(g)   Some females just seemed to really like each other, such as the pair Blondie and Ardith, and the mother and daughter duo Gray and Zira described in the chapter: *Mothers and daughters.*

Chimpanzees in the second region of dense rain forest in the Taï National Park in the Ivory Coast were of another race (*Pan troglodytes verus*). Christophe Boesch and Hedwige Boesch-Achermann (2000) concluded after 15 years of chimpanzee observation there that the females built strong friendships among themselves, groomed each other, took an active role in social conflicts against males, made alliances, chose males with whom to have sex, and supported their sons long after they reached adulthood (see the chapter: *Mothers and sons, and providing free food*). These chimpanzees also differed from those at Gombe because they had a more forested habitat and were never provisioned; it had taken longer to habituate the animals to their presence, but the researchers knew that their animals' behavior had not been skewed because of the free food, which caused fights and a shift in the community's home range (See the chapter: *Mothers and sons, and providing free food* for a discussion on provisioning).

These researchers report that high-ranking females were often members of a bonded dyad, unlike low-ranking females. These bonded pairs, which were usually about the same age so unlikely to be sisters, formed alliances in conflict situations and shared meat when it was available. The authors cite the friendships of Ondine and Salomé who were seen together 66 percent of the time over an 18-month period,

Malibu and Poupée seen together in 71 percent of sightings during this period, and Loukoum and Gauloise seen together in 79 percent of sightings. These pairings lasted for five, five, and four years, respectively, before the death of one of each pair. The slightly older Ondine was the alpha and Salomé the beta female of their group. Even when Salomé was in full estrus with a large pink rump swelling, and followed all day by the adult and adolescent males of the community anxious to mate with her, her very close friend Ondine was there too, along with the offspring of both of them. The authors note that in the Gombe research area adolescent females sometimes remained in the community and, thus, mothers might form close friendships with their daughters as did Fifi and Flo, and Passion and Pom (see the chapter: *Mothers and daughters*). However, in the Taï forest, chimpanzee females reaching puberty all emigrated from their group to join another. Each of these newcomers, by combining her interests with those of another female, increased her power within her new society. Friendship for Taï female chimpanzees develops when they come together as adults to form a community, and they become highly socialized in the process (Lehmann and Boesch, 2008).

Boesch and Boesch-Achermann believe that differences in behavior among females seem to depend on two demographic factors: community size and adult sex ratio. When the community is small, such as that in the Taï National Park (its size reduced dramatically by disease and human predation), a larger proportion of the community members will comprise each group or party that is briefly together. This means that males and females are likely to be present in each group. Taï also had a greatly skewed sex ratio, likely because of poaching, with relatively more females compared to males than in other communities. For both these conditions, it would be fruitful for females to have partners join them in an alliance to ensure power within the group. The fission–fusion system allows group members to adapt flexibly to the community situation; social systems can vary in one population over time and in populations living under different conditions.

MOUNTAIN GORILLAS

I had not expected to find special friendships among female gorillas, knowing that most females emigrated from their natal group and joined another with unfamiliar individuals (Watts, 1994). However, females in a mixed-sex troop (which includes all of them, as females are never alone or in all-female groups) do occasionally have preferred partners with whom they spend time, sitting or lying in contact, and grooming together (Bagemihl, 1999). Females have sex with each other, even those who are heavily pregnant, but some dyads are especially likely to be together as favored partners. To initiate sexual activity, one female approaches another, making copulatory vocalizations, after which they sit together quietly. They then begin to fondle each other's vulvas with their hands or mouths, which leads to a face-to-face embrace, usually while lying down. This leads to pelvic thrusts and rubbing their genitals together, often while making "growling, grunting, screaming, or pulsing whimpers." Sometimes one partner will pause to caress the other, shift her position, or masturbate herself. These sessions are, on average, five times longer than sexual encounters between a male and a female. In these, the male thrusts against the female from the rear, with few displays of affection such as embracing and grooming.

BABOONS

Baboons behave as the emigration hypothesis predicts: the sex that remains in the natal group, in this case females, will be the one with close bonds. Shirley Strum (1987) notes that friendship ties between two olive females (*Papio cynocephalus anubis*) are often strong enough to last a lifetime. There are looser bonds between males and females as we saw in the chapter: *Male and female pals – not just for sex!*, but only short-term alliances between two males.

Peggy and Constance were best buddies, almost inseparable. Peggy was a favorite of Strum, the highest-ranking female in the troop she was observing. Her youngest infant Paul was next in the line of hierarchy, followed by the next youngest in a reverse order of age. Her behavior helped Strum figure out the basic organization of the troop. Wherever Peggy was, there too was Constance, both feeding, resting, and walking together. Strum had wondered when she first knew them if they were sisters, as they were too near in age to be a mother and daughter. But they could not be sisters, because Peggy was the older and dominant. Over the years that Strum watched them interact, the two remained grooming partners and companions, calm, and relaxed. If either was in a conflict, the other supported her. Constance, although high-ranking herself, benefited more from Peggy's help and her dominance than vice versa. However, Constance's presence could sometimes tip the balance enough to ensure that Peggy would not lose a battle with an adult male.

Because they were about the same age, their youngsters grew up together, although family demands sometimes trumped their friendship. When Peggy's family was especially large, she had less time to socialize with Constance – there are only so many hours in the day. Constance did not seem to mind though, because their fellowship continued in its own gentle way. It did not preclude camaraderie with a male because old Sumner, the male Friend of both of them, was content to sit about in a threesome with offspring playing nearby.

Years later, perhaps inspired by Strum's findings, three women researchers, Joan Silk, Jeanne Altmann, and Susan Alberts (2006a), decided to do a huge, thorough analysis of friendships: with what other females did each female baboon (*Papio cynocephalus*), living in seven study groups in the Amboseli Basin of Kenya, form special friendships? Documentation had been kept on the activities of 118 females from 1984 to 1999, including which pairs were involved in joint grooming and the identity of neighbors within five meters (16 ft) of each individual, recorded at one-minute intervals; these two items of grooming and proximity, if frequent, were defined as reflecting special bonds between dyads. The data set was voluminous, comprising 5690 hours of observation during which a total of 1430 dyads of females lived in the troops at the same time. The female dominance hierarchy was calculated from watching incidents of aggression between two animals (it remained remarkably stable over the years), the maternal relationships of the animals was known from long-term genealogical records, and the paternity of many of the baboons was determined by DNA samples from blood and feces.

Many of the dyads had weak social bonds but a few had remarkably strong friendships. Bonds were strongest among maternal kin, especially between mothers and daughters (who have half of their genes in common), and then maternal sisters. Less favored were maternal aunts and nieces, maternal cousins, paternal kin, and non-kin (with fewer genes in common). Whether or not a female's mother was present or absent was important; maternal absence strengthened relationships with maternal sisters and weakened relationships with maternal aunts. When few maternal kin were available to a female, she began to strengthen her bonds with paternal sisters. (With such findings one begins to ruminate about relationships within one's own extended human family!). These facts are, of course, not cut and dried. Not all friendships can be postulated from an animal's relatives, particularly when dominance and age are of some importance (friends tended to be of similar age and dominance). No female had a very large social network (perhaps that would have required too much time to be feasible), and it is nice to report that most females had at least one tight friendship with another female, even if there were no close maternal kin in her group. The researchers conclude that "The social lives of female baboons revolve around a tight core of close associates with whom they form stable and equitable relationships."

In a paper discussing further aspects of the same research project, the same trio of scientists (Silk *et al.*, 2006b) worked out, for each female, her top three most friendly partners, judging from the proximity and grooming present in each dyad, for each year separately. In any given year, X might have been one of Y's top three partners, but Y may not have been one of X's; however, this was not usually the case. The most equitable grooming relationships occurred between females from the same maternal lines which were either close in age or close in dominance rank. The 14 dyads that groomed the most equitably also tended to form the most long-lasting bonds. Among the baboons which had close bonds lasting at least five years, five pairs were mother–daughter dyads, five were maternal sisters, and three (and perhaps the fourth) were paternal kin. Other social bonds lasting at least three years were present in 13 pairs of true non-kin, so that inheritance was not everything. Some dyads end because one partner falls ill, is eaten by lions, or grows old. The partner then may find a new mate, perhaps a sister or a daughter who has grown up. The authors conclude that "The capacity to form and maintain strong, equitable, and enduring family ties and friendships, as well as more opportunistic relationships, may provide long-term benefits for female baboons."

These researchers emphasize that female friendships where there is female philopatry (females remaining in their natal territory) are important for various reasons (Silk *et al.*, 2006a). They:

- reduce levels of aggression among females,
- increase care for dependent young,
- decrease the cost of maternal investment, and
- reduce the risk of infanticide.

The reproductive success of each female depends on her longevity and on the survival of her infants (Cheney and Seyfarth, 2007). How long a mother lives is often a matter of luck (as predators and disease can attack at any time), but the survival of her young depends on her ability to form relationships with other females and with a few males to protect them. Her hierarchical ranking is not especially important, because even the lowest-ranking female regularly produces offspring. Baboon females in Amboseli with the highest lifetime reproductive (and therefore evolutionary) success were not those who ranked highest, but rather those who were most socially integrated in their groups (Silk *et al.*, 2003).

Friendships have been vital in the evolution of baboons. Close social bonds are highly adaptive, but it is impossible for any one individual to bond closely with dozens of others. In Amboseli National Park, females had between no and six close bonds with other females, with an average of 1.6 bonds. Either females do not have enough time to become close buddies with more females or they do not need a very large number of friends to meet their social requirements (Silk *et al.* 2006a,b).

JAPANESE MONKEYS

Because extensive grooming is important in friendships between Japanese monkey adults (*Macaca fuscata*), various studies have focused on this activity in these animals, which live in large troops comprising both males and females. Grooming between two female buddies is by far the most common. During five months of observations of allogrooming, Naoki Koyama (1991) found that among the 42 adult females, 17.5 percent of possible pairs formed grooming partnerships, grooming 784 bouts in total; dyads of females related to each other groomed the most. Between heterosexual dyads there were only 129 grooming bouts, with most of these duos being related and females doing most of the work. Among the eight male adults, only one pair groomed each other, and only two times. So social grooming among females is significant in this species, although in this study we are not given information about any two individuals who were especially friendly.

Over a decade later, Masayuki Nakamichi (2003) published research showing that as wild female Japanese monkeys at Katsuyama, Japan, grew older, they spent less time grooming with unrelated individuals, especially if they were low-ranking, but kept up this activity with kin. He discovered this, in his record-keeping of grooming activities, by dividing the 83 wild females into five subgroups, three relating to age (5–9 years, 10–14 years, and 15–22 years) and two to high- or low-ranking of the females. Unlike the low-ranking females, the high-ranking females attracted as many unrelated monkeys to groom with them as did the younger high-ranking ones. Why might females change their grooming activity with age? Nakamichi suggests two reasons. First, with reduced energy because of her age, an older female will need to cut back on her grooming, and prefers to groom only with relatives. Second, females like to allogroom with individuals of about the same age; as she grows older, a female's friends begin to die off so she has fewer chums with whom to interact, but a continuing number of younger relatives. Eiko Kato (1999) had shown earlier that females like to keep close with kin as they age, especially if they are high-ranking. These high-ranking individuals were popular with non-kin not only for grooming, as we have seen, but also for proximity.

Female friendships in this species can last for at least ten years. Masayuki Nakamichi and K. Yamada (2007), who had carried out research on females grooming each other in a free-ranging group of Japanese monkeys in 1993, decided to do the same thing ten years later to see if and how partnerships might have changed over this time. They had 18 adults who were still alive to consider, ranging in age from 17 to 32 years old. On average, in 2003 each female groomed with 2.2 partners she had groomed with ten years before, with 3.5 partners related to these surviving partners, and with 4.5 partners with whom she had not groomed earlier. Of course, the possible number of grooming partners was large, including all other monkeys in the troop, so the authors worked out statistically the likelihood of particular partners being chosen. They found that the 18 monkeys in question were generally conservative. They had concentrated their grooming interactions on closely related females, on some unrelated females such as surviving old partners, and on some females who had been related to these old partners. However, they had also chosen a few new partners with whom to groom, indicating a liberal tendency. Some females abided by a similarity principle, grooming with unrelated females who were similar to them in dominance ranking and/or age. Long-term psychological bonding between pairs could be impressive. One female had been fairly high-ranking until she fell to the bottom position, yet she still maintained a grooming relationship with her higher-ranking friend, three years older. Two other unrelated females of the same age but with very different ranking positions had also kept a balanced grooming partnership (grooming each other about the same amount of time) over the ten years.

Japanese monkey females maintain social connections with gentle vocal "coo" sounds as they feed or move in groups. This way, individuals keep in touch with each other over a distance when they are out of sight. For his research on Yakushima Island, southern Japan, Masazumi Mitani (1986) taped, over two months, the "coo" sounds of the 12 adults of M-troop (comprising three matriarchal kin-groups), both those emitted and responses to them. Computer analysis could identify the voiceprint of the vocalizers for two-thirds of the adults, and it seems likely that all the monkeys could recognize each other's calls. His results showed that the three matriarchs exchanged frequent "coo" sounds with each other, that the other females exchanged these sounds with the females in their kin group, and that the males were little involved in such exchanges.

BLUE MONKEYS

How friendly are blue monkeys (*Cercopithecus mitis*)? Each group comprises many females but only one male, who has no male associates with whom to interact; when several females are in estrus at one time, other males may invade the group for copulation, something the resident male cannot physically prevent, so he certainly is not fond of them. The females have grown up together but they often like to be alone, perhaps feeding or resting, so research had to be carried out over a long period to collect enough data to determine if they had any special friends at all among themselves. Marina Cords (2002) did this over a period of 21 years. She found that in the Kakamega rain forest of western Kenya, the social bonds of the monkeys (who are not actually blue except for a bluish tinge to their faces) were so weak that each spent on average less than five percent of their time during daylight hours in social activities such as grooming or sitting beside one another. However, they did care with whom they associated; in one study group, the average female groomed with only seven of the 14 partners available. Typically, the time spent grooming with a preferred partner was at least ten times greater than the time spent grooming with the least favorite female, and a few dyads groomed together much more often than did other pairs. Some females were within one meter (3 ft) of their favorite partner 100 times longer than they were with their least favored partner. Reciprocal egalitarian grooming occurred mainly after the females had combined forces to fight any groups that infringed on their territory, which incorporated their food supply, and they did this as if to reinforce their collaboration. Then they spread out to enjoy the rest of the day by themselves.

HORSES

Sociality is the basic characteristic of horses; each wants to be with other horses or, failing them, other herd animals such as bison. When

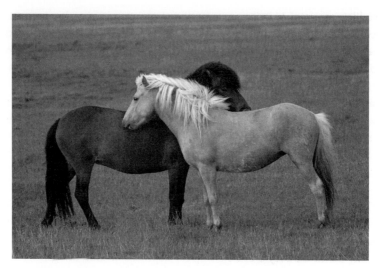

Figure 2. Mares form a close bond through allogrooming.
© Anne Dagg

horseback riding and camping, one usually needs to tether only one
horse, as long as it is the right one, which is the lead mare (Rees, 1997).
All the other horses, including the stallion, will stay with her. Frank
Dobie (1955) relates a story that in 1820, a solitary mustang followed an
expedition in the American West and hung about its campsite that
evening after the men's horses were staked out. It was as if any company were better than none. In the morning, however, he was shot for
food. It is horses' sociality that has enabled humans to take advantage
of them and bring them into bondage. When domestic horses are kept
in isolated quarters, they suffer from not being with their own kind.

Robert Vavra (1979), who was well acquainted with free-ranging
horses in the Camargue marshes of southern France and in Spain (kept
mainly for the Spanish military), reports that friendship bonds were
often strong in female herds. Best friends could almost always be found
together, one often resting her head on the other's back, a sure sign of
camaraderie. Once when a mare became separated from her herd, she
and the other females reacted in a panic bordering on hysteria, neigh-
ing and galloping about as if berserk. On another occasion when a third
female tried to edge into the affections of one mare of a dyad, the other
rushed toward her, biting and kicking the intruder to chase her away.
Jealousy and possessiveness were the emotions most in evidence
among female herd members. In small mixed-sex herds, the band

stallion's insistence in keeping all the females together and away from other males tended to eclipse such bonds; the male himself often had a favorite mare with whom he associated and groomed during quiet times (Rees, 1997).

When two mares form close bonds with each other, their friendship is cemented by grooming sessions: the more friendly a dyad, the more they groom each other. Mutual sessions begin with a horse who wants to be groomed approaching another (Vavra, 1979). If the other is agreeable (judging by her ear, eye, and body response to the proposition), the animals stand together for a few minutes, smell each other's nose and neck, then position themselves head to tail beside the other. They then give short, firm bites at each other's mane and neck, areas which they cannot reach on their own bodies, untangling hair and removing dead skin, their activity often audible from a distance. From the neck, they work their way back with their teeth along the shoulder and back, stopping at the tail root. Sometimes the mares then change places and begin grooming on the other's second side, starting again with the mane. While they are at work, they may swish their tails, dislodging and shooing away horse flies and other bothersome insects from their buddy's face (Morris, 1988). The sessions do not take long, lasting usually three minutes at most, nor are they only about cleanliness. Allogrooming is also a symbol of belonging to a group and having a special companion within that group. For this reason, horses should be groomed routinely by their human companions, preferably their riders, to tighten the bond between the two. The deep friendships that people have made with horses are discussed in the chapter: *Animal and human "friendships"*.

While many horses pair up to become best friends, others form a spontaneous dislike of another for no apparent reason, an antagonism which may fester for years. Desmond Morris (1988) notes that "horses housed in groups, in fields or paddocks, will soon start to display all kinds of idiosyncratic preferences for particular companions." There is a rough dominance order in a group (for example, the subordinate mare usually instigates grooming while the dominant one generally terminates it), but this tends to be superseded by the bonds between close dyads. However, in truly wild horses there is little or no female dominance in that resources such as grass and water are usually unlimited.

Two so-called Judas horses in the Cedar mountains of Utah were best buddies (Morin, 2006). They had been taught to lead wild herds into traps after they had been rounded up from overcrowded areas; then they could be captured and adopted into human families. The mares were a pair of bonded registered thoroughbreds: "They were just in love with each other." One was kept in a home corral while the other was released at one of the wings of the trap just before wild mustangs were herded past. They tended to follow her into the trap as she rushed to be with her sister. She hated to be locked in with the wild horses, though, so she would kick madly at the gate until she was let out and could rejoin her buddy.

The Icelandic horse is a wonder, a sturdy animal with long flowing mane and tail emblematic of its island home. Icelanders are so proud and protective of these animals, originally brought to the island by Vikings about 1000 years ago, that no other horses are allowed into the country in case they corrupt the native breed. If an Icelandic horse leaves the island, it cannot return (Bunge, correspondence from Canadian Icelandic Horse Federation, 2009, Jan. 23). Hrefna Sigurjónsdóttir and three colleagues (2003) decided to find out how semi-wild Icelandic mares (aged ten to 19 years) would behave if there were no bossy mature stallion to keep them in line. Their research involved watching a herd of 34 animals over a five-week period, day and night (because there is no real night in May and June when the research took place). Half of the herd comprised mares which had been together for most of their lives, all in a linear dominance hierarchy; the rest, all subordinate to the mares, were geldings or subadults. The watchers monitored the horses from an observation hut inside the 200 hectare enclosure or from outside the fence so that they would not disturb them. The activities recorded included allogrooming between two individuals and the presence of play, when horses chased each other in a friendly fashion or play-fought. Every half hour, a map was made of the position of each animal so that preferred associates could be calculated; later, a circle on the map was drawn around each individual to ascertain the heads or tails of which horses, her special friends, were within two horse-lengths of her. This measure represented the personal space and the individual flight zone of a horse. The results of the research were calculated from 488 hours of observation and 534 maps.

Although each horse had total freedom to go anywhere in the huge enclosure and consort with any other horse, the mares formed their own closed herd, leaving the geldings and subadults to join together in a second, inferior group. One basic difference between the groups was that none of the mares played, while all the horses in the second group did. Aggression among the mares was slight, occurring perhaps only to keep the dominance hierarchy in place. Preferred or special friends were defined as those who spent much of their time close together and groomed each other often. The pairs of mares who allogroomed most were close in rank order and, since rank was correlated with age, similar in age. In addition, the closer they were in the dominance hierarchy, the more related they were. Popularity among the horses was impossible to predict from observations, however. All horses had at least one preferred friend, but most had three or four; only Drífa had seven. Drífa was sixteen years old and ranked eleventh in the dominance hierarchy, so her attractiveness was not obvious from the data.

What did the absence of a stallion mean for the group of mares? Most obviously, the mares groomed more and had more preferred partners than they would have had were a stallion present. They also groomed mostly with each other, rather than with their weaned offspring. In the absence of such maternal attention, the offspring tended to bond with their peers and with the adult geldings. With a herd stallion absent, adult females took over stallion behaviors, such as mounting females in estrus (this happened 47 times) and protecting a foal.

Foals born into a band of free-ranging horses leave it when they reach puberty to seek breeding opportunities elsewhere; their mothers, who are unrelated to each other, remain stable members of the band. Elissa Cameron and two colleagues (2009) wondered if females living in New Zealand formed special friendships with each other and if so, whether such friendships affected their behavior. To this end they recorded the activities of 55 feral females along with stallions. Over a four-year period, for each mare as a focal animal, they tabulated for an average total of 38 hours, (a) all mutual grooming between her and another mare, (b) whether she was closer than two body lengths from another mare, and (c) whether she had initiated this closeness. They also noted how many foals each mare produced and whether each lived to be at least one year old – the measure of each mother's reproductive success.

After analyzing the three values measuring what the researchers called social integration for all the mares, they found that significantly more young were born to females with a close friend than to females without. This result was independent of the quality of the habitat, social group type, dominant status, or age. A mare might be pestered by males or other females, but this harassment decreased if she had a close buddy. If there were more than one stallion in a band, females had fewer offspring and were more protective of their foals, perhaps for fear of infanticide. In primates, special friendships are usually correlated with kin and therefore have a genetic base, but in these unrelated horses, there was a direct benefit through their number of young for the mares who had a close friend.

ZEBU CATTLE

Behavioral studies of domestic animals often focus on aggression within a group because this could be a problem for the farmer or rancher. If their animals fight each other, they might lose some of their commercial value through wounding and stampedes. This emphasis on aggression is a pity because almost all interactions among domestic herd animals are amicable. The team of Viktor and Annie Reinhardt (1981) decided to study relationships in a herd of zebu cattle (*Bos indicus*) comprising one adult bull and 30 cows living on a large ranch on the Athi Plains of Kenya. The kin relationships of the animals were not known. The researchers observed the cattle under natural conditions for three years, and then for several more years after some of the animals were removed. Aside from being yarded at night to prevent predation, the zebus were not castrated, dehorned, or milked, and were free to interact with each other as they wished. The human observers walked among the herd taking notes, keeping 1.5 meters (5 ft) away from standing animals and 0.5 meters from those lying down so as not to disturb them; sometimes they took movies of activities. The zebu were never more than about 160 meters (175 yd) apart, so they could all be seen at one time.

The friendly behaviors noted by the Reinhardts were "social licking" (when a cow licked a partner in a body region she could not reach herself) and "social grazing" (when from two to four cows kept close together while grazing for at least half an hour). "Preferred partners" were defined as those who licked each other or grazed together most often, while an individual's "associates" were those recorded as being preferred as licking or grazing partners (these were usually not the same) for three or more consecutive years.

The results of the study were clear cut, showing many cows preferring to graze with and to lick other specific individuals year after year. These pairs were obviously good buddies. Alma was the most popular cow, preferred by six others in grazing associations although she herself preferred to graze with two of them especially, Dora and Monika. As the dominant female and leader, when she decided to move somewhere else, all the others followed her. She was similar to them in age, reproductive history, weight, and social rank status, but she had attractive qualities that made her herd-mates watch her constantly. Four other pairs were also preferred grazing partners (one cow could have several of these), but 17 showed no preference for a connection with any particular cow and were themselves not preferred by any other female. In all, 12 of the 29 cows (one died) had preferred special grazing partners over three years.

As noted above, licking associates were not usually the same as the grazing associates – only five cows chose the same partner for both activities (which seems strange in human terms. If you had a friend you wanted to eat beside and you liked licking, why not lick her and be licked by her?). But even stranger, whereas two mares groom each other reciprocally, in the 20 cows which formed a licking association (some had two partners), 19 had one cow always licking the other, while only one had a mutual or reciprocal licking association. Twelve cows did not lick any other cow preferentially, while 20 cows were not licked preferentially by any other cow. Daisy was the preferred licking recipient for five cows, but she did not lick any of these or any other cow preferentially. What made Daisy so attractive as a lickee? The Reinhardts were not able to figure this out. She was not a leader like Alma and she seemed, in every way, no different than her sisters. Of the 29 cows, 24 had a preference partnership of some sort with at least one other cow. Only three individuals had a particular partner whom they preferred for both activities: for example, Gilla and Nanette were each other's long-term favorite associate, not only for licking but also for social grazing.

The researchers analyzed the grazing and licking propensities of calves born to the cows, which do not concern us here, but they did find that partnerships were formed in young calves of about the same age, and that by the fifth year, such male–male partnerships were waning while female–female partnerships were not. Apart from special friends, siblings were the second preferred grazing partners of all calves in the herd. The closest pair was twin heifers who, for 52 consecutive months, preferred to graze with each other rather than with any other calf. No calves had any preferred licking partners, however.

The Reinhardts discovered in their research that close friendships (as defined by grazing or licking) were important among the cattle, could last five years or more, and occurred between both relatives and non-relatives. Taken altogether, 83 percent of the cows had at least one other buddy in a relationship that lasted for at least three years. Most of the cow partnerships were probably founded on sibling attachments, on earlier friendships between unrelated calves, or on mother–calf bonds. However, although most cows were popular with some colleagues, a few did not have a single close friend. The evidence suggests that female calves grow into cows which tend to stay near their mothers, even as adults with their own young. The Reinhardts conclude that in natural cattle herds the social structure is "based on matriarchal families which in their turn are interconnected by means of friendship relationships between non-kin partners."

The lone bull of the herd has not been discussed here. He showed no preference for any of the females beyond copulating with those in estrus who wanted his services. He had two sons who grew up as buddies until one overthrew the other to succeed his father as the boss animal; from then on, the other began to avoid him, so they were no longer friends.

Among domestic groups of cows (as well as of pigs and sheep) many individuals who have grown up within a group continue to spend time together, share food, coordinate activities, and allogroom (Hatkoff, 2009). They share an easy comfort with their pals. When such friends are separated, their heart rates and levels of stress hormones increase, they learn less quickly, and they are less resilient, becoming more frightened of new situations.

LIONS

Lion cubs are born into an incredibly social, polygamous environment. Initially, they live with their mothers in a safe den, and then with other mothers and young about the same age in a pride. If their mothers are away on a hunt, they can suckle from the female who has stayed behind to be with them. They have endless time to play and explore as they grow. In his aptly titled book *My Pride and Joy*, George Adamson (1986) writes at length about his wife Joy, and their great friendship with lions, especially the famous Elsa. He notes that this communal upbringing sets the stage for bonding between contemporaries within each sex when they reach adulthood, which is vital to their way of life. Males become such close comrades with one or a few other males that if they manage to join a pride, they will willingly defer to each other in mating rights (see the chapter: *In brotherhood*). The females who have known each other since birth continue to be close buddies, who now form efficient hunting parties to bring down large prey as food for the pride.

Unrelated females may become fast friends too, as the Adamsons found when they brought together orphaned and other young lions to form a pride of 16. Arusha, who was sent to them as a cub from the Rotterdam Zoo, and Growlie, from a Nairobi orphanage, became as close as sisters, even though they had been born on different continents. When they put radio collars on some of their lions, they only needed to collar either Arusha or Growlie, not both, as the other was always near her friend. (A tight male friendship also formed between Leakey, a Nairobi orphan, and Freddie, a cub whose mother had been killed hundreds of kilometers away. Although they were a year apart in age, a collar had only to be put on one of them, because the two would always be in the same place.)

In her book *Lions Share: The Story of a Serengeti Pride*, Jeannette Hanby (1982) describes the amazing closeness shared by the nine young females making up the Sametu pride. Lion prides comprise sisters, cousins, nieces, aunts, grandmothers, and even great-grandmothers, but the Sametu pride females were all about the same age and therefore full sisters, half sisters, or cousins. Hanby calls them all sisters, and these close friends spent most of their time together, playing, grooming, resting in a heap, rubbing against each other, or licking faces as they relaxed, their cubs romping or wrestling among them, the mothers allowing other youngsters as well as their own to suckle. Sometimes a female might crawl under another to encourage the other female to mount her (Bagemihl, 1999); then the mounter would act out behavior associated with heterosexual mating – nipping her partner on the neck, growling, making pelvic thrusts, and afterward rolling about on her back. Then the two friends might reverse their roles.

The pride females were usually only apart for two reasons: when each new mother chose a secluded place to give birth and hide her newborn cubs until they were old enough to be introduced into the pride, and when they were hunting, sometimes going off in ones or twos to catch small prey (Hanby, 1982). There was strength in numbers should unwanted males attack, as well as great pleasure in fellowship. Females of all ages were equal, with no leader among them. They only competed with each other when they were hungry and feeding at a kill; food was sometimes hard to come by when each female needed over five kilograms (11 lb) of meat a day.

Hanby and her researcher husband, David Bygott, spent four years at the Serengeti Research Institute observing this pride, making a card for each individual, which showed the face outline, any ear notches, and permanent black whisker-spots on both sides of the muzzle, so that they would always recognize him or her in the field. The cards also noted special features such as a tail tuft missing (Safi), a distinctive scar (Sega), or missing teeth. Each lion was given a native name beginning with S to reflect their membership in the Sametu pride. Research on lions in this area of Tanzania had originated with George Schaller who founded the Lion Project in 1966; it was carried on by Brian Bertram from 1970 to when Hanby and Bygott arrived in the mid-1970s. At first, Hanby and Bygott had no idea where the pride of nine females came from, but by checking the notes of Bertram, they realized that they had all been born to females in the Masai pride in the prolific year 1971, three and a half years earlier. They had left their natal pride when neither the new males nor their mothers wanted them around because there were newborn cubs to rear. The females were used to humans hanging around them making notes, so they were fairly tame.

George Schaller in his book *The Serengeti Lion* notes that some females spent more time together than others. For example, in 1967 A, B, E, and F were often together, the first two with cubs and the last two, older, without. In a triad, elderly lion C hung out with young adults G and H when all three had young cubs. The following year after E had died, B and F became rather solitary while A teamed up with H and I. C, G, and H were still together, joined often by I. Seven females, who had cubs in late 1968, formed a tight group for the next six months – most were seen by Schaller on 66 days, on 55 of which all seven were present together. Females who had young cubs of about the same age tended to hang out in a group, their youngsters playing together as if on a human play-date. Such relationships often remained strong even if the cubs died. Other close friends wanted to be together not because of their cubs, but because they liked each other's company. Female subadults might be forced out of a pride if it were becoming too large, but no foreign female ever joined one (Schaller, 1972).

SPOTTED HYENAS

Bloody Mary, the clan matriarch, her beta friend Lady Astor, Mrs Brown of more humble status, and Old Baggage were four spunky female spotted hyenas (*Crocuta crocuta*) who lived in the Ngorongoro Crater of Tanzania in the 1960s. Jane Goodall and her husband then, Hugo van Lawick, came to know them well in the years they spent filming and watching predators near the Den of the Golden Grass that the hyenas called home (van Lawick-Goodall and van Lawick-Goodall, 1970). About 60 hyenas belonged to the Scratching Rock clan that Hans Kruuk (1972) had studied earlier, one of eight territorial clans present in the crater. Many of the hyenas in this clan were recognizable by sight by such anomalies as a blind eye, scarring on the body, a gimpy leg, or by posture or way of moving. Because the spotting pattern on each torso is distinctive, each hyena also had his or her photograph taken from either side for identification purposes.

In this social species, females are dominant to males; they defend their clan territory, visit and use communal scent places, and hunt, just as do males (Kruuk, 1972). Best buddies Bloody Mary and Lady Astor, followed by 18 clan members, led one attack against two hyenas from the neighboring Lakeside Clan who had had the temerity to settle down at their territorial boundary. One of these interlopers was fatally wounded by the Scratching Rock hyenas before the growls, screams, and whoops filling the night air attracted even more hyenas from both clans to battle. Again and again Bloody Mary, Lady Astor, and their team were forced by the enemy to retreat into their own territory before they regrouped and surged forward again in a frenzied, noisy attack. Twenty minutes later, a truce somehow prevailed as the clan members separated to return, some bleeding and limping, to the core of their own territory.

Periodically, a "marking party" comprising Bloody Mary, Lady Astor, and other clan members reinforced their territorial boundary by sniffing out and replacing a scent mark deposited by one of the neighboring clan, perhaps on a stalk of tall grass. After they had each jostled forward to smell it, Bloody Mary carefully positioned the stalk between her hind legs beside her protruding scent glands and moved slowly forward, leaving behind a strong-smelling secretion. Lady Astor repeated the process after Bloody Mary had stepped aside, followed by other clan members. Then the group loped off along the boundary line to repeat this rite many times.

Near the Den of the Golden Grass in the core area of the Scratching Rock Clan, various cubs spent their long childhood, older juveniles played, and adults relaxed during the day. There Bloody Mary had installed her two cubs, Vodka and Cocktail. (Jane Goodall gave them neutral names because it was difficult to tell the sexes apart, with the females' enlarged clitoris resembling a penis. Several times she had to change the name of a supposedly male animal when it gave birth to offspring.) Lady Astor had an older youngster there too, whom

Goodall had named Miss Hyena because one day she was seen peering into a pool of water at her reflection.

Fast friends Bloody Mary and Lady Astor did almost everything together. Each weighed a solid 59 kg (130 lb) and, given the vast number of prey animals in the crater, they and their followers were able to kill game almost every night. After each kill, they hurriedly stuffed themselves to repletion in case lions happened by, Bloody Mary claiming the head as her alpha right. She could easily break open the skull with her strong teeth and jaws to get at the brain. Once the group feasted on the carcass of a wildebeest, which had somehow tumbled into the Munge River. Bloody Mary took the time, when she came to the surface to breathe and wolf down a chunk of meat, to move her paws about to ascertain the body's exact position in the muddy water. The hyenas around her who did not do this tended to come up empty after each dive. Because of their rough diet, the hyenas periodically coughed up hair balls on which they loved to roll.

The two close friends made sure that everyone knew they were in command. This included mobbing, with a few hyenas attacking a clan mate for no apparent (to humans) reason. Once when Baggage was sprawled at the Den of the Golden Grass, peacefully suckling her twins Sauce and Pickle, the duo and another female approached and stood over her, growling and biting her shoulders and back. Baggage crouched down, squealing, before slinking off to a site nearby with her screeching cubs in tow. She was mobbed there again and forced to move, and then mobbed a third time before being left alone. Bloody Mary and Lady Astor also took it upon themselves to prevent some females from mating, sometimes rushing at a copulating pair to knock them apart.

Baggage was old and medium-ranking in the hyena hierarchy, as was her best friend Mrs Brown. These two hung out together just as Bloody Mary and Lady Astor did, although their meals were not as fresh. Once they and their cubs tackled a dead hyena, Old Gold, whom lions had killed but not eaten. It lay in the sun for a day and had been rolled on by cubs before the two families finished off the rotting remains. Baggage and Mrs Brown often spent the heat of the day in the cooling mud of a reed bed not far from the Den of the Golden Grass that held their two sets of twins. By late afternoon they roused themselves, covered in slime, to return to their young. At the den mouth they gave short, low-pitched calls to their cubs who came scrambling up into the open air to greet their parents. Baggage's cubs were each quick to latch onto one of the two teats of their mother who lounged at the den entrance. There they leisurely sucked for an hour or more as the sun set. Because hyena mothers do not take their cubs to a kill, nor bring back meat to the den, they suckle them for eighteen months or more until they are able to feed themselves.

On one such communal nursing occasion, a pride of lions came sniffing over to the den to see what was available. Baggage, Mrs Brown, and Bloody Mary, who were all suckling their young, gave warning growls to their cubs who immediately disappeared into the den; then they fled to a safe distance to watch what would happen. Dens used by hyenas have small, extra cavities dug out by the cubs where they can hide from predators such as lions or even hyenas; the latter are cannibals, which is perhaps why the female hyena is larger and dominant to the male and therefore better able to protect her young from male attack. The lions knew that the cubs were there, but fortunately for them and their mothers, did not bother to try to dig them out.

GRIZZLY BEAR

Often there are brief records of close buddies that whet one's appetite to learn more. Such was the friendship between two female grizzly bears (*Ursus arctos*). Brothers Frank and John Craighead (1972), world experts on this species, in one study in Yellowstone National Park put radio collars on two females whose movements they were following via their radio signals. All during the summer of 1966, bear No. 40 with her two cubs was fast friends with bear No. 101 and her cub. They stayed as if *en famille*, hunting for food, resting, sleeping, the youngsters playing together, until the families entered separate dens in the fall to begin hibernation. Presumably to be near her friend, No. 40 did not den where she had previously, 26 km (16 mi) from the den of No. 101, but instead chose a site only 2.5 km (1.5 mi) away. Until winter conditions became too severe, the families visited back and forth between the dens as if reluctant to end their summer relationship. All other bears and bear families that the researchers had monitored had sought solitude before hibernating.

The following spring, the two-family alliance became even stronger. No. 40 weaned her yearlings, went into estrus, and mated with a male while No. 101 kept her yearling and adopted those of her friend. The Craigheads note that this change was beneficial, because one of the two females would be producing offspring a year sooner than usual, and the three youngsters would still have two mothers to protect them during the summer. The authors do not report what happened next in the life of these families.

Bruce Bagemihl (1999) reports on other pairs of female grizzlies who were best friends but not, as far as was known, sexual partners, traveling and feeding together with their cubs during the summer and fall seasons. The four cubs responded to either mother equally and occasionally suckled from both. The two mothers jointly defended any food they killed or came across and protected their young from predators, including male grizzlies. Should one female die, the other usually adopted her cubs, caring for them along with her own. In one 12-year study, close bonds between two females occurred during four of these years. About nine percent of grizzly cubs were raised in families with two co-parenting females.

BOTTLENOSE DOLPHINS

For seven years David Lusseau and his colleagues (2003) studied the bottlenose dolphins (*Tursiops* sp.) living in Doubtful Sound, New Zealand, in the extreme south of this species' worldwide distribution. This fjord is an unusual habitat for dolphins in that the water is deep, coastal, and geographically isolated; there is virtually no emigration or immigration of individuals in this dolphin population. The researchers wanted to figure out the organization of the dolphin society, which differed from that of dolphins elsewhere. To identify individuals, they photographed each one and named him or her on the basis of natural markings, shape, size, or scarring of the dorsal fin. They ascertained the sex of an animal by using an underwater videocamera mounted on a pole.

The 83 known dolphins of Doubtful Sound lived in large mixed-sex groups. Unlike in other dolphin populations, some of the females did have a complex network of female friends, defined as individuals present together more than one would expect if the distribution of the individuals were random. A female who had a number of preferred companions was also likely to be the one who gave the "upside-down lobtailing" display in which the dolphin rolled onto her back, exposing her ventral surface to the air, and then slapped the water repeatedly with the dorsal side of her tail. This was the signal for the group to stop traveling (Lusseau, 2007). (The "side flopping" signal, in which a male, usually, cleared his body entirely from the water and landed on his side, was a display activity that indicated that the group should begin to travel.)

The researchers' results showed that some close associations among females lasted for at least seven years. This meant that these friendships were not affected by the birth of young, unlike in Florida's Sarasota Bay where groupings are more fluid and females change their association pattern after giving birth to maximize protection of their calves. On the east coast of Scotland, too, associations between individual dolphins were far more likely to be short-term than in the Doubtful Sound population. Shifting relationships allow information about the availability of fish to travel quickly through the social network of a population, which would be desirable if fish numbers were patchy or changed rapidly within a season (Lusseau *et al.*, 2006). A few male–female associations were also stable for at least seven years, something unknown in dolphin populations elsewhere (Lusseau *et al.*, 2003). These could not all have been mother–son relationships, because some males had more than one female associate. Doubtful Sound also had male–male associations, which are common in dolphin society.

The authors argue that the unusual social organization of dolphins in the Sound may reflect the low biological productivity there. Survival may require a greater level of cooperation than for dolphins that live in more productive places, and this may have determined the group stability. They write that dolphins, as a top predator, may "need to possess information on the location of food resources in time and space that can only be gathered over several generations." Thus, it may be that acquisition of food has shaped the social organization of the dolphins. It would also explain why males and females have long-term associations that are not necessarily involved with reproduction. Group stability is, of course, connected to the isolation of the population in the one fjord. The researchers conclude that the social plasticity of the species as represented by the Doubtful Sound population "is an important factor in this species' ability to exploit an extraordinary variety of habitats."

BALEEN WHALES

Baleen whales such as gray, blue, right, bowhead, and humpback whales live not on fish, but on krill and other planktonic crustacea, which they strain from the water by means of horny baleen plates hanging down from the sides of their upper jaws. Their food is so dispersed that none of these species live in very large groups; instead, they travel alone or join a few others to migrate or gather food in biologically productive areas. Usually it is difficult to know if they are present together because of sociality, or because that is where the food is (Connor and Peterson, 1994). Whales make vocalizations that travel long distances in the ocean waters, so although a single animal may seem to be alone, he or she may in fact be in fairly constant contact with other whales of which the human observer is unaware. A large number of these individuals are transients who are not seen together later on, but some may form friendships; humans have killed millions of dolphins and whales over the centuries, but intensive research on cetacean behavior only began in the early 1970s, so there is a huge lack of information about them.

The behavior of humpbacks (*Megaptera novaeangliae*) is better known than that of most baleen whales. Females tend to hang out in small numbers where there is food, but males, who are intolerant of each other, keep apart and are often alone. Theirs is a fission–fusion society, like that of bottlenose dolphins or chimpanzees, in which all the members are not present together at any one time. In the Gulf of Maine, where humpbacks are studied as they slowly migrate each year back and forth from their tropical breeding grounds to the arctic where they obtain most of their food, female associations are clear during the two-month observation periods and these often continue annually during the whales' summer visits (Connor and Peterson, 1994). For this species, therefore, some females form friendships that last for years.

LAYSAN ALBATROSS

This albatross (*Phoebastria immutabilis*) seems a model of monogamous bliss each November at the small colony at Kaena Point Natural Area Reserve, Hawaii where, after six months of solitude soaring on two meter (6.5 ft) long wings over the Pacific Ocean, individuals finally return to their breeding site. They seek out their mates so they can settle down to produce and incubate their single egg for 65 days, and raise their nestling. These birds can live for 60 or 70 years, a long time to enjoy a bonded life. When she was the first lady of the United States, Laura Bush praised these couples for making lifelong commitments to each other (Mooallem, 2010). What a good example for human beings! However, what Bush did not know because the males and females look alike, and what could not be known until recently with DNA analysis, was that the pairs were not necessarily male and female; almost a third of the time, they were two females. The birds in Oahu only began re-colonizing sites in 1992, after a severe population decline of the species in the 1970s. The number of females coming to the colony increased faster than the number of males (59%–41%), so that often two females formed tight bonds; one such female pair has lasted for at least 19 years.

To make sure that there could be no mistake with the sex determination, Lindsay Young and two colleagues (2008) tested the DNA of feathers from all of the birds in the colony up to four times; there was no doubt that many of the couples comprised unrelated females who had had sex with a variety of either paired or unpaired males. About half the time, each of the females laid her own egg, but only one was incubated and subsequently hatched. This nestling was related by blood to only one of the females, but even so, theirs was an egalitarian relationship with full cooperation between them in raising their chick.

All the albatross couples not only looked alike, but as parents they also behaved in the same way, incubating the egg in turn and both bringing food for their voracious infant. Heterosexual and homosexual couples had equal reproductive success in raising their young, although problems with incubation meant that the female pair were less likely to have their egg hatch; the homosexual pairs were therefore not as productive as the heterosexual ones, but had they not chosen to pair up with their mate, they would have had no young at all. In long-established colonies that have an equal number of males and females, most couples will be heterosexual, but for female–female couples who joined together initially to raise their young, their friendship apparently remains firm for the rest of their lives.

As we have seen in this chapter, females of many species form friendly pairs for a variety of reasons: allogrooming, aggressive coalitions, sex, support for blood relatives, protection of offspring, sharing food, sharing nursing (lions), facilitating the entrance of immigrants to a group (bonobos), having infants act out play-dates; but surely also the pleasure of companionship.

In theory, adult males in a group should be rivals, each determined to mate, because of his evolutionary destiny, with any female who comes into estrus. In reality, males in many communities may actually be best buddies, as we shall see in the following chapter.

In brotherhood

Male animals are far less likely to be bonded in male–male friend-ships than are female dyads because, at heart, male priority is to mate with females. Males are therefore usually rivals. However, most females only mate when they are in estrus, which never lasts very long, so male friendships may blow hot and cold. For example, adult male blue mon-keys (*Cercopithecus mitis*) sometimes groom each other and hang out with particular friends, but this easy companionship exists only when there are no females around. The same is true of patas monkeys (*Erythrocebus patas*). In species in which males and estrus females are present together in a group, males are typically antagonistic or, at best, grudgingly tolerant of each other (Kappeler, 2000). In such groups the biggest, most aggressive males tend to have the most success with females, so males have evolved to be larger than females (Neuhaus and Ruckstuhl, 2002). Male primates may form coalitions to attain power for some end result (for example, combat against another group), but these are ephemeral in nature and do not usually last. Human brothers and male relatives are often close friends but so, too, can they become enemies. About 1800, ruling sultans had a tradition of fratricide, where brothers, nephews, and any other threats to ascendancy were generally imprisoned and killed (Nagel, 2004).

This chapter considers friendships among primates (chimpan-zees, gorillas, Tibetan macaques, and woolly spider monkeys), horses, lions, cheetahs, wolves, bears, dolphins, and birds (geese, rheas, black swans, Humboldt penguins, and long-tailed manakins).

EAST AFRICAN CHIMPANZEES

It must be difficult being a male chimpanzee. How to balance a commit-ment to his friends, his community, and his own needs? Unlike females, most males live in the same group for their whole life, at different times experiencing both high tolerance of, and intense competition toward fellow males. Their prime role is to join together to keep their territory and the group females and young safe by patrolling the border and fighting, even to the death, any invading chimpanzees. They also form short-term coalitions to achieve some aim, such as organizing hunting parties to capture young antelope or monkeys to eat, or arranging a group attack on alien chimpanzees. The adult males form the stable core of a chimpanzee community, although these members may spend relatively little time together because of their fission–fusion lifestyle.

To illustrate the ups and downs of male chimpanzee friendships, Goodall (1986), from her work at Gombe, notes the history of Figan and three other males. Figan was friendly with his older brother Faben as they grew up, but this friendship was shattered when he challenged Faben and became dominant over him. Figan was friendly with Humphrey and Evered toward the end of their lives, but hostile toward them earlier, confronted with issues of rivalry about mating with females and the dominance hierarchy order.

Grooming is important in fostering friendships, with male chimpanzees spending more time on this activity than do less amicable female duos or male–female pairs (Nishida, 1990); grooming between two males strengthens a pair bond and may be correlated with such things as support in acts of aggression and/or the attainment and maintenance of a higher dominance rank (Watts, 2002). Michael Simpson (1973) researched grooming behavior in 11 adult males who frequently visited Goodall's feeding site to obtain bananas. Simpson found that individuals had preferences about whom they chose as a grooming partner, although this was difficult to measure quantitatively because individuals came and left the feeding site at different intervals, and stayed there for varying periods. Oldsters Mike and Goliath, for example, always groomed each other when they were visiting the feeding site at the same time, while other pairs never did so. Goliath was the most enthusiastic groomer with the longest overall median grooming duration of ten minutes. Those males with the highest status were most involved with grooming, especially with receiving it.

In 1981, Yukio Takahata (1990b) studied relationships including grooming among six prime males over twenty years of age and four younger adults, in the Mahale Mountains not far from Gombe. He observed that the two most dominant males, NT and BA, scarcely associated with each other (although they would form an alliance years later), but instead were the centers of two separate clusters. Each comprised three lesser males who gave NT or BA pant–grunt barks (as a submissive chimpanzee does to a more dominant one), often stayed close to them, followed them about, and groomed with them. NT and BA groomed other prime males more than they were groomed themselves (unlike Simpson's important males), while the younger adult males tended to groom among themselves. Takahata found that there were stable friendships between three male dyads: NT and LU, MU and LU, and BA and DE. (NT was an exceptional male who held the alpha position of his group for at least ten years. He often groomed other chimpanzees and allowed older males to share his meat, but he was fiercely aggressive in attacking strangers.) It seemed that although the alpha male changed his preferred friends now and then, he usually associated with older males who were declining in the dominance hierarchy. In this way, he did not encourage up-and-coming younger males who might become his rivals in future (Kawanaka, 1990).

What about a male's own needs? Each male wants to be dominant to demand respect from other chimpanzees and have first access to sparse commodities such as meat and, if he can organize this, a consortship with a female in estrus. Copulation is rare for chimpanzees because females only come into estrus about every four years. Sometimes a dominant male can persuade a sexually receptive female to go away with him as a consort so that he alone mates with her, but at other times she succeeds in enticing many males into copulation; Goodall's friend Flo, when she was about 40 years old and in estrus, mated 50 times in one day with an assortment of males (1986). Of course, the males in a group are related to each other, so all had at least some genetic input in the infants born into the group.

To improve his status, a male has to challenge and fight those in the dominance hierarchy above him, his erstwhile friends, and he has to ensure that males subordinate to him are kept in their lowly place. Depending on conditions, the relationship between any two males will tend toward a fluctuating association of positive, neutral, or antagonistic interactions; it is a conundrum that males vie with one another to build and maintain supportive relationships with individuals whom they cannot trust, and who cannot trust them, because each is bent on pursuing his own selfish interest. On one hand there is equality between animals when they play, groom, and share food; on the other there is inequality in that the dominance hierarchy as well as age means that some individuals will benefit at the expense of others (Takahata, 1990b). A couple might be grooming each other and sharing meat tidbits one week, then fighting over alpha status the next.

Nicholas Newton-Fisher (2002) studied 12 adult male chimpanzees of the Budongo Forest in Uganda who lived in a community with three adolescent males and 14 females, collecting data over 15 months on grooming, number of pant–grunt vocalizations, proximity of individuals, and acts of aggression. He found that each prime male was seldom alone, but with at least one other male over 90 percent of the time; each had about seven or eight individuals with whom he hung out, but he definitely preferred some males to others. In a large group, he associated with preferred individuals while avoiding others.

Does the environment affect sociality? Perhaps, as we saw for female chimpanzees in the chapter: *In sisterhood* who were fairly friendly toward each other, thanks to the large natural food centers where they congregated for most of their meals. (As a food source, these fruiting trees cannot be compared to bananas provided by researchers which, because they were limited in number, could cause fighting – see the chapter: *Mothers and sons, and providing free food* on provisioning.) Although all males had conflicting aims as we have seen, those from the forests of Uganda seemed to be more friendly toward each other than those of Gombe and the Mahale Mountains in Tanzania, where large food trees were lacking (Ghiglieri, 1988; Newton-Fisher, 2002). Close friendships may develop in old age, however; seniors Mike and Hugo in Gombe eventually put their years of squabbling behind them to be replaced by a peaceful, companionable, joint retirement (Goodall, 1986); the old males Leakey and Mr Worzle, whom Goodall met early in her studies, had a very close and supportive relationship too, but their earlier history was unknown. (Pairs of old animals will be discussed in the chapter: *Old buddies.*)

MOUNTAIN GORILLA

Adult male mountain gorillas (*Gorilla gorilla beringei*) either wander by themselves when they leave a troop, join a female or two to become a one-male group, or hook up with an all-male troop (Robbins, 1995); there is no possibility of joining a group that already contains both sexes because of intense competition among males for mates (Yamagiwa, 1987) although, rarely, a grown-up son may continue to live in his natal group (see the chapter: *Fathers and sons, and social grooming and preening*). Joining up with other males is an odd choice biologically because there is no chance for reproductive activity. It is in these all-male troops, formed when the females leave a troop or solitary male gorillas join forces, that close friendships are fostered between individuals, many of them sexual in nature (Bagemihl, 1999). All-male groups, which may persist for years, have a complex network possibility of homosexual couplings. Males have a preferred partner or, rarely, up to five partners with whom they have sex. Sometimes an older male courts and "guards" a young favorite to prevent advances from other members of the group.

Juichi Yamagiwa (1987) gives an example of behavior in a troop of six unrelated, mature and maturing males in the Virunga mountain gorilla population, including the silverbacks Peanuts and Beatsme[1] made famous by Dian Fossey in her research. The animals remained together as a cohesive group for over three years – their daily activities of foraging, traveling, resting, and playing highly synchronized and the members physically as close together, or even closer on average, than gorillas in mixed-sex groups. Over the three months he followed this group, Yamagiwa recorded all interactions between its members as well as noting their distances from each other, at ten minute intervals. Despite the group cohesion, tension among the members based on jealousy over homosexual partners led to considerable aggressive behavior, with individuals changing their preferred partners often during the months. Fights were usually directed by an older male at a younger one, although Peanuts and Beatsme had eight major bouts in which they wrestled, bit each other, and suffered various injuries. During homosexual behavior, the older males usually competed for and mounted the younger ones, perhaps implying that the silverbacks considered themselves as "owners" more than friends such as are present in female bonobo societies. Yamagiwa concluded that for younger males, being in an all-male troop may, at the least, protect them from the hazards of lone travel or other misfortunes as they mature.

Courting activity involved one male approaching another with intense panting noises until they were touching (Bagemihl, 1999). This led to mounting and thrusting by the active participant, which might occur in either a front-and-back or, more often, a face-to-face position while the two involved emitted growling, grumbling, or panting sounds. After ejaculation, the instigator broke free with a deep sigh. These sessions, like those between two female gorillas, lasted longer than male–female copulations. With the exception of the two silver-backs who only mounted, the others took turns in either of the two positions. Bruce Bagemihl reports that male gorillas in general appear less interested in sex than females, who almost always initiate hetero-sexual activity.

A bond between two brothers may extend into a lasting friendship, as proved to be the case with Makale and Mutesi who lived in the Bwindi Impenetrable National Park of southern Uganda. These two adults were familiar to Thor Hanson (2008) who served as an American Peace Corps member for two years from 1993, in charge of habituating a wild gorilla family to the presence of people so that a local tourist industry could be implemented. This family contained a female, an alpha male, and five other males, so Hanson was not surprised when Makale and Mutesi decided to go in search of greener pastures. He had noticed in the months before their departure that the two had spent more and more time together, often moving at the edge of the group, harassing the younger males and, for Makale, terrifying Hanson and the African trackers. As a duo on their own, Makale and Mutesi wandered about the Park, presumably hunting for females willing to leave their family group. When they came near their old family, the alpha male backed off so as not to cause a confrontation; had he lost the battle, he might have lost his only female as well.

Twelve years after he had left his position as a gorilla minder, Hanson returned on a visit from America to Bwindi. The trackers told him that his old nemesis Makale had continued to terrorize gorilla families in the area until, eventually, a female had joined him. He had then chased off his older but less aggressive brother Mutesi and set up his own family group, along with a second female adult. Hanson was able to count the family's most recent night nests – for Makale, two females, a juvenile, and one infant. A happy outcome for Makale, if not Mutesi.

TIBETAN MACAQUES

Hideshi Ogawa (1995) set out to study the curious bridging behavior of males among Tibetan macaques (*Macaca thibetana*), a behavior reported also for several other species of macaques living in multimale–multifemale groups. Bridging involved two adult males simultaneously lifting up an infant between them, often sucking or touching its genitalia in the process, and then grooming each other. One male would come forward with the baby, which they would gently raise between them, one lifting up its shoulders and the other its hips, while the infant lay on its back forming a bridge between them. The baby's mother would observe her youngster's elevation with equanimity; she had mated with most males in the group and was correct in believing that her youngster would not be harmed. Bridging activity was presumably important because it developed and maintained friendly relationships between the males, but otherwise it seemed very strange. Previous researchers had suggested two reasons for it. One was that by handling a baby, subordinate males reduced the possibility that they would be attacked by dominant males. The second, called the baby-sitting hypothesis, was that related males held up the infant thereby informing each other that this was a relative of whom they should take special care in the future.

If the first agonistic buffering hypothesis were true, then one would expect: (a) that males likely to be attacked would handle infants more frequently, (b) they would handle them in situations in which they would be most likely to be attacked, and (c) they would be less likely to be attacked while handling an infant. If the second baby-sitting hypothesis were true, (a) males would use infants who were related to them for bridging and would have friendly interactions with them, and (b) males would provide benefits for the youngsters.

To solve this puzzle, Ogawa watched one group of Tibetan macaques at a feeding station and in the nearby forest in Anhui province of China over many months, for a total of 1173 hours. These monkeys had been the subject of research for years, so that the male linear hierarchy and many of the females' relatives were already known. During his research, Ogawa observed and recorded bridging behavior between two males and an infant 333 times.

The data indicated that the agonistic buffering hypothesis was the correct one for several reasons. It was usually subordinate males, for example, who carried an infant to a more dominant male with whom to form a bridge, apparently as an appeasement effort to reduce social tension. If the second male refused to handle this infant, the two males were less likely to groom each other than if he did – bridging activity was never followed by aggression, but often by allogrooming. There was a positive correlation between the frequency of bridging and that of social grooming, indicating an affiliative behavior between the two males. The baby-sitting hypothesis was not supported because natal males did not prefer to handle infants of their own matrilineage compared to other infants. In addition, young males and new immigrant males who had rarely copulated with adult females in the preceding mating season also had bridging interactions with infants, although they were very unlikely to be related to them.

In primate species in which groups contain a number of adult females and males, the males often do not get along well because of tension over mating opportunities. Perhaps bridging behavior, given the warmheartedness that so many adult male as well as female primates feel for infants, has evolved in some macaques to tamp down male aggression within a group. Infants are useful in other species, too, for a social purpose. For example, bridging somewhat resembles the holding of an infant to his chest by one male baboon during an encounter with another male, hoping in this way to reduce the possibility of an attack by the second male.

WOOLLY SPIDER MONKEYS OR MURIQUIS

Karen Strier and two colleagues (2002) carried out a ten-month study in Brazil on friendships among groups of male woolly spider monkeys (*Brachyteles arachnoides hypoxanthus*); they chose this species because, unlike in most species, males do not have a dominance hierarchy, do not become rivals during the mating season, and do take turns copulating with females in estrus.

These spider monkeys live in fairly small groups, and small groups are all there are to research because few members of this highly endangered species still exist in the wild. Karen Strier (1992) had been the first to study the behavior of this species, specifically the Matão troop (initially composed of 23 animals, which later grew to 42), one of two troops on an old coffee farm in south east Brazil near the Atlantic Ocean; the owner had carefully preserved the forest habitat where they lived.

Are things necessarily as they seem? From the results of their research, they note that male duos were often fast friends, spending lots of time together and even mating with the same receptive female. Yet the research also showed that two sets of brothers with the same mother were *not* particular friends, even though they shared many of the same genes, which seemed odd. But let us look at the research itself.

The lack of aggression within a group is correlated with their large size – nearly 15 kg (33 lb) for both males and females. They live mostly in the high forest canopy where they feed and through which they travel fast, using their prehensile tails; they have evolved not to fight because there is too much of a possibility of being hurt or killed in a fall. One can imagine pugnacious individuals picking fights over the years and tumbling out of trees now and then, leaving their more peaceful relatives behind to reproduce more pacific youngsters like themselves. If two woolly spider monkeys want to eat at the same fruiting site, one will wait his or her turn or move to another branch rather than confront the other. Because the males and females are about the same size, the females cannot be pushed around by the males.

The research involved watching and following one individual at a time for ten minutes, noting down his activities (feeding, resting, traveling, socializing, or "other") minute by minute, his embraces with other monkeys, and who was in physical contact with him, within one meter (3+ ft) and within five meters (16 ft) of him. Each male was observed for an average of 26 hours during the study. Any other events were recorded as they occurred, importantly 123 copulations between specific males and females.

These males were fairly social – on average, each spent 55 percent of his time near at least one other male, far more of his time than he spent near females (19%), although there were more adult females (18) than males in the troop. Males do have preferred male friends: dyads that were friendly with each other were more likely than other males to mate with a particular female, and certain males embraced each other more – 76 percent of all embraces seen were between males and functioned, in part, to repair friendships after rare spats.

Males were especially likely to stay close together when the group was resting, a period when most copulations occurred. The researchers wondered if they stayed near each other then, not because they were friends, but because they wanted to be around other males to monitor their mating behavior in case one detected a female in estrus. If one did so and copulated with her, she would probably mate with them too. Males do not battle each other for mating opportunities as in many species, but take turns copulating with the lusty receptive females, as often happens in chimpanzee groups. Competition does occur, but it is among the sperm of the mating partners; the larger the volume of sperm implanted by a male into a female's vagina, the more likely he is to father a female's next infant, although the timing of mating with the period of ovulation is also vital.

The case of maternal brothers was somewhat baffling. In the group, there were two such fraternal sets: DA and DI were prime males aged 10 and 14 years, while NE and NI were a young adult male of 9 years and a prime male of 14 years. Theoretically, one would expect brothers to be more amiable than usual because they share many of the same genes. Yet DA and DI were among the ten male dyads who never embraced each other, while NE and NI only embraced once. However, each male of a set was friends with another male (RB and BLK, respectively), with whom he shared copulation partnerships and a close friendship, judging by their proximities. These brothers usually traveled in the same subgroups, although they did not stay close together and rarely interacted. The researchers postulate that perhaps there was no need for them to reinforce their relationships by hanging out together or embracing, because they had overlapping social networks to alert them to the reproductive condition of females. In this way they could gain their reproductive ambitions indirectly.

Strier and her colleagues found that males developed distinctive styles of friendship. The mature male CL, for example, was the most social, spending 80percent of his time with at least one other male and forming strong pair friendships, but he had a very low maintenance rate, meaning that it was usually other males who approached him to be together; he was highly tolerant of males attracted to him. By contrast, the much younger RB, who was almost as social (with 76 percent of his time near other males), had the highest maintenance rate of any male in the study; he was responsible for sustaining ten of his 12 dyadic associations, four of which were with much older males. Young adult males often had special friendships with mature males, the former usually taking the initiative in approaching his pal. The researchers suggest that perhaps the young adults are attracted to seniors because they are especially tolerant, have a greater ability to detect estrus in a female, and tend to be chosen by females as mating partners because they are experienced.

This study was a fascinating one, but of necessity left many questions unanswered. Do males really associate with each other to increase their chances of mating, rather than from simple friendship? Do males try to time copulations so that they occur when the female is most likely to be ovulating? If the mature males had fathered some of the young males, were they aware of this and might it have affected their joint behavior? Were there paternal brothers in the group? If so, did they know of their relationship and behave differently because of it? Even the socializing of 13 animals among themselves can be endlessly complicated.

HORSES

Because of their social nature, horses want to be with other horses with one notable exception: most band stallions loathe rival males. Wild mustang stallions in the American West always stay with their family group to make sure their mares are protected; they perceive other males as competitors, not possible buddies (Dobie, 1955). All the males without families, including the juvenile, the old, and the mediocre, belong to bachelor groups that do not include females; these males are often close friends who play-fight or groom each other during rest periods. But why do some of these mustang bachelors form dyad bonds while others do not? Why do hyperactive horses tend to link up with docile, submissive ones? Robert Vavra (1979) suggests that age, temperament, and friendship between their mothers are probably important. While they last, bachelor pair-bonds can be very intense, with fights for possession of a friend as violent as those over the chance to mate with a female.

Bachelor bonds usually break down if one of the pair becomes a dominant stallion with his own family of mares and their young. One exception was the band stallions Endo and Findo of the sociable Fjord breed, who had grown up together (Schäfer, 1975). Sometimes they brought their separate bands to the same pastureland in the morning, where the two friends would groom each other at length during their mid-day rest period while their females and young intermingled peacefully.

Claudia Feh (1999) studied the behavior of horses in the Camargue area of southern France where, in 1974, 14 horses of known genetic background had been released into a pasture of 300 hectares (750 acres) comprising grasslands, freshwater marshes, and salt steppes. By 1980, the number of horses had increased over six-fold, so some were removed regularly after that to prevent overgrazing. All the animals were tame enough to be readily approached, were known individually along with their birth dates, and had had their blood taken to identify their fathers.

Feh, who observed the horses from 1976 to 1987, focused in part on the social lives of long-lived stallions in one herd. These males were in sight of each other most of the time, and all wanted to mate with females. How did they go about this without constant friction? To answer this question, Feh first spent two years working out the dominance hierarchy of the males by noting head threats, bites, rearings, and kicks between pairs of animals: who gave them and who retreated from them. This required between 564 and 1872 hours of observation of each stallion. Occasionally, she cut off the water supply temporarily so she could stimulate increased amounts of aggression among the males who crowded into the watering area. At the same time as she was working out this hierarchy, she was noting at 15 minute intervals which males stayed close to which other males, again accumulating mountains of data on individual preferences.

When young colts were first evicted by the band stallion from the family in which they were born, they joined an all-male group. Soon afterward, some of them tried unsuccessfully to monopolize a female, although it was not until they were four years old that they would be ready to mate. Other pairs gathered together a few females between them, but later split because each male wanted a family group for himself. This desire was feasible and accomplished by three high-ranking stallions, but not by the low-ranking ones. To Feh's surprise, some of these young males would forge two-male family alliances in future; they were already becoming close buddies with each other in the male group.

Of the 13 stallions in Feh's focus, four of the low-ranking males developed close bonds with another low-ranking male, initiating permanent family groups that contained not one but two stallions. One of these pair-bonds lasted for at least 16 years. The two stallions who set up a family together were each other's closest associates. They groomed each other often, the activity initiated usually by the subordinate male. (Grooming reduces the heart rate of a horse when directed at the lower neck area, where a major nerve ganglion under the skin is located [Feh and de Mazières, 1993]). They also sniffed at each other, had frequent body contact, and sometimes gave gentle agonistic rank displays that caused no physical harm. They were about the same age but not more related to each other than to other herd males. If there were an intruder near their family, both males might confront him, or the subordinate one might do so while the dominant male, who spent most time with the females, rounded them up to keep them from the stranger.

What were the benefits and costs for the two stallions in their family group? The dominant male had a partner to help with fights that occurred year round – indeed, the subordinate male fought competitors more than twice as often as did his friend. (Feh compared the coats of two white stallions with reverse melanism – the hairs on their body grew in black where there was a scar from a fight. When they were 20 years old, the stallion that had his own family group had 35 permanent scars whereas the subordinate stallion from an alliance had 146.) The subordinate male benefited because he was able to sire about one-quarter of the foals born into the family; he would have been less reproductively successful if he had had to adopt a "sneak" mating strategy as other non-band males did. Benefits for both were a high survivorship of their foals because the family had two males to defend them: only three percent of neonatal foals in two-male families died compared to 22 percent in one-male families. Why so many foals died was unclear, but a number of them were wounded accidentally soon after birth by brawls among adults. There was no evidence of deliberate infanticide. In summary, in general low-ranking males have little access to females in estrus, but they can overcome this deficit by forming an alliance and friendship with another male that can last their entire lives.

Hans Klingel (1998) has studied the behavior of the closely related African ass (*Equus africanus*) in the Danakil Desert of Ethiopia and the Asiatic wild ass (*Equus hemionus*) of the Karakum Desert in Turkmenia. Unlike the domesticated horse, both species live in unstable groups of variable composition in their dry environments, with no indication of permanent bonds between any adult individuals.

LIONS

George Schaller, the first zoologist to study lion behavior in depth, found that pride males (*Panthera leo*) have a tight bond. They may be brothers or cousins born about the same time and reared in the same pride, or they may be unrelated males who met as nomads, became familiar with each other, and teamed up together. Rarely can a lone male become a pride male because he will be defeated in battle by larger male groups. Even fairly large groups will only retain the status of pride males for a few years before they are deposed by younger and stronger males (which prevents incest between a male and his grown daughters). The bond between pride males is not necessarily genetic, but always that of familiarity and congeniality. Pride males seldom fight seriously among themselves (the possibility of injury would be great), nor do they compete for mating opportunities with a female in estrus once she has accepted one of them. If one male begins to copulate with a female, his companion will wait (if he has a day or more to spare, because mating courtships can last up to 55 hours [Schaller, 1972]) until his friend is satiated; then he himself can hope to mate with the female if she is still willing, which she often is (Packer *et al.*, 1991). This tolerance seems strange at first, but indicates how strong the friendship bond can be among pride males; if an unrelated lion allows another male to copulate instead of himself, he may forfeit his own chance to be a father and to pass along his DNA to the next generation. However, statistics show that male lions in groups of three or more, compared to males of one or two in a pride, can hold onto a pride longer, mate with more females, and produce more infants who survive, so that each male has a higher reproductive fitness because of their cooperation (Bygott *et al.*, 1979).

In her book *Lions Share*, Jeannette Hanby (1982) describes six brothers, born about the same time in the Loliondo pride, who left that pride to seek their fortune in 1971, the same year in which the females of the Sametu pride were born (see the chapter: *In sisterhood*). One died, but the other five were soon mating with members of the Masai pride, and then with members of two other prides as well. Such males are democratic, without a hierarchy, as we have seen, and without any one animal acting as a leader. They are, like the three Musketeers, all for one and one for all. Together the Loliondo males defended a territory comprising all the prides or parts of prides that included their cubs and the females who bore them; in effect, they acted as ranchers who owned a large territory in which lived prey animals to provide them with food and females with whom to mate and reproduce.

Despite their psychic closeness, the males were often apart from each other, enjoying days-long mating sessions with females in estrus – Brian Bertram (1978) calculated that pride males he radio-tracked spent one-fifth of their time copulating![2] – as well as patrolling their real estate, marking their territory borders with sprays of urine, or relaxing with groups of females and cubs. When they did come together, united by roars that enabled them to find each other, their shared greetings were exuberant: rubbing faces (there are glands above the eyes), sliding their bodies along each other to exchange individual scent, perhaps one falling against another and toppling him to the ground where they rolled and lolled about (Hanby, 1982). Sometimes the greeting was so intense that after caressing between a pair, one male mounted the other complete with thrusting movements (Schaller, 1972).

Resting pride males sometimes groom and lick the mane of a pal after a rainstorm to dry it or imbibe the fresh water. Grooming made their manes look larger, which might intimidate non-pride males, but nevertheless acted as padding against attacking claws or teeth. However, the very size of their manes made hunting by stealth difficult for their conspicuous owners. In order to eat well, males had to join females around one of their kills, forage on opportunistic kills, or scavenge (Hanby, 1982). On reading Hanby's book, I was unable to determine if any male dyads in the Loliondo pride were more likely to interact in a friendly way than were other dyads; they were all good buddies together.

Two other males observed by Hanby and her husband David Bygott did form a close dyad: Kesho and Kali (Hanby, 1982). They left their natal pride together, as two-year-olds in 1971, to become nomads, wandering about to find what food they could muster and careful to avoid territorial areas defended by aggressive pride males or females.

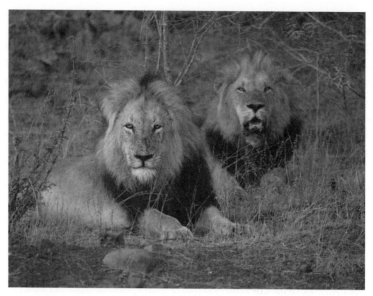

Figure 3. Male pride lions are friends for life.
© istockphoto.com/Jonathan Heger

When they rested, they licked each other's head, neck, and shoulders. They were seldom apart, the only friend each had. By 1973 they had joined the Nyamara pride; two years later they were with the larger Sametu pride where they mated with all nine females. They remained together and with this pride until 1976 when Kali disappeared, at last breaking up their seven-year friendship. Kesho stayed with the Sametu pride for a while by avoiding the Loliondo males, but was finally chased away by them the following year. He became a nomad again, but this time a solitary, friendless one who disappeared in 1978, fate unknown.

CHEETAHS

Although cheetahs (*Acinonyx jubatus*) are usually depicted as solitary animals whose forte is running down medium-sized mammals to catch and kill for food, sometimes several cheetahs team up together. Most common are pairs or even trios of adult males. Initially these males were assumed to be brothers, but by checking the spotting on the animals and referring to long-term records giving their history and parentage, Brian Bertram (1978) found that some were unrelated. Pair-mates, who may remain together permanently, spend almost all their time together, defending each other in fights, resting while physically touching and often grooming by licking each other's faces (Bagemihl, 1999). If they are separated, perhaps during a lengthy chase of prey, they become upset, giving loud chirpy calls so that they can find each other again. Once reunited, they display great affection, purring, rubbing their sides together, and sometimes mounting each other, having erections. Two males should be able to chase down larger prey than a singleton could, and to encroach on the territory of a solitary male; one battle of a pair of male cheetahs attacking and defeating a solitary male has been filmed.

Cheetahs in Africa are far less common than in the past, but at least some are not too stressed by the increasing number of tourists anxious to see them. Bertram reports that not only do they sit on termite mounds to have a better view of their surroundings, but once habituated to the presence of people, they sprawled comfortably on the hood of his landrover for the same purpose. Groups usually consist of a mother with her cubs, but rarely two females will join forces, sometimes an anestrus cheetah mounting the other if she is in estrus, clasping her partner with her forelegs, gently nipping the scruff of her neck, and thrusting against her (Bagemihl, 1999).

WOLVES

Wolf packs (*Canis lupus*) are hierarchical in nature, so it is amazing that a high-ranking male should choose the omega male to be a close buddy. Yet this is what happened in the wolf pack that Jim Dutcher put together in order to film two best selling documentaries: "*Wolf: Return of a Legend*" and "*Wolves at our Door.*" The first title reflects the fact that Dutcher settled his pack in the Sawtooth Mountain range in Idaho where wolves had become extinct many years earlier, driven out or killed by settlers, hunters, and farmers. The second title was appropriate because Jim Dutcher and his wife, Jamie, built a yurt for themselves in a small fenced area within the fenced ten hectares (25 acres) where the pack lived. For years they spent most days observing and filming the behavior of the wolves around them, so their book *Wolves at our Door* (2002) is full of details about how the animals interacted.

One fascinating discovery was that the beta wolf, Matsi, was a devoted friend of Lakota, the omega wolf. Matsi was the brother of Kamots and Lakota, who had been born a year earlier. His name was the Blackfoot word for "sweet and brave," which depicted his character well. Kamots (named in Blackfoot for "freedom") was the alpha male, dominant to all other pack-mates, and Lakota (named ironically with the Sioux word for "friend," when he was to have so few) the omega male, subordinate to all males including the cubs as they grew to adulthood. Matsi seemed content to be second in command because he did not have the confidence or aggression of Kamots, nor of course the shyness and deference of Lakota. Lakota had been the loser in the series of dominance fights that had convulsed the pack early in its formation, resulting in his lot in life: becoming the scapegoat and focus of the pack's aggression. The role of the beta wolf is more vague than that of the alpha or omega animals, and for Matsi involved patrolling the pack territory, taking care of the pups, and maintaining peace and order. The beta animal usually takes over the alpha role if the alpha male is killed or injured, but he must not seem to challenge the alpha animal, nor must he be too overbearing with those under him, in case he does become head wolf in the future. Matsi was gentle most of the time although, as a yearling, he had helped his pack-mates force his older brother Lakota into omega-hood. As he continued to adulthood, however, he became a peacemaker.

The Dutchers only realized that Matsi was a good pal to Lakota when they went over their slow-motion films, frame by frame. In one series of shots of Kamots and Matsi (the two top wolves) feeding on a deer carcass, Lakota tries to pick up a bit of meat that has been tossed aside. Matsi growls and chases Lakota back a meter. Another hungry male then attacks Lakota too, but Matsi attacks this male and knocks him off Lakota. Matsi is chastising the male who was disciplining Lakota for not knowing his place. On another roll of film, the pack was mobbing Lakota for some infraction, all trying to hurt him, when Matsi burst into the throng as well. The Dutchers at first had assumed he was jumping into the melee to help harass poor Lakota. Looking carefully through the "blur of fangs and fur," however, they realized that he was, in fact, body-checking one attacker and inserting himself between Lakota and his tormentors so that Lakota could escape.

Matsi and Lakota were so closely bonded that when the wolves spread out to rest, Matsi and Lakota often slept side by side. If Matsi went exploring, Lakota joined him. They often played together, Lakota enchanted as they chased each other and fought mock battles, because he did not have to worry about Matsi suddenly turning on him in anger for some slight. The Dutchers could not find any good reason for this unlikely friendship. Certainly it was wonderful for Lakota, who had no other friend and who might benefit from some protection. But Matsi had lots of friends. Did he understand what a horror being an omega must be, and at times willingly try to lighten Lakota's life? Matsi did have standards, however, and Lakota was never allowed to interfere with his meals. On one occasion, Jim Dutcher saw Matsi approach Lakota, lift his leg and urinate over his back in response to some transgression, but later that day they were playing together again and they slept side by side that night.

In August 1966, for political reasons the Dutchers were forced to leave the pack, but they remembered the wolves with love and affection and had movies documenting their behavior. One man who watched their films said that he used to hunt and kill wolves, but after seeing them on the Discovery TV channel as social animals with a close family life, he would never do this again. Strangers throughout North America told the Dutchers that the adventures of Matsi, Lakota, and Kamots had changed their way of thinking about wolves. This is a worthy heritage.

BEARS

Adult male bears usually travel alone, but not always. Among polar bears (*Ursus maritimus*), adult males "fairly commonly" travel together not because there is any reason for their alliance but because they obviously like each other (Ashworth, 1992). Additionally, sibling American black bears (*Ursus americanus*) who have been abandoned by their mother because she will soon be expecting a new family sometimes stay in contact with each other for two or three years, well into adulthood, traveling, feeding, and even denning together. Benjamin Kilham (2002) suspects, from his years of work with black bears, that friendship or mentoring between males, as well as short-term friendships outside the breeding season between unrelated males and females without cubs, may be common.

BOTTLENOSE DOLPHINS

Few large species are harder to research than ocean mammals. Richard Connor and two colleagues (1992) spent 25 months studying the social behavior of male dolphins (*Tursiops aduncus*) in Shark Bay, off the coast of Western Australia, but conditions were frustrating. They were not always sure if the 300 individual animals they could finally identify in dolphin schools were male or female. They had no idea which individuals were genetically related, or of a dominance hierarchy among them. Sometimes males were aggressive toward females, but at other times a male would help a sick schoolmate by supporting it so that it would not drown. The researchers never saw an actual copulation, yet they soldiered on and were able to report that many pairs and triplets of males are indeed closely bonded.

The researchers were fortunate in their choice of location for their work. At the Mama Mia campground in Shark Bay, 850 km (530 mi) north of Perth, up to a dozen dolphins have been hand-fed by people in the shallow waters near the beach since at least the early 1960s. By using small boats, the scientists could survey the familiar dolphins that haunted the shallows as well as those farther out. They became well acquainted with the "tame" dolphins and, with the aid of visual sightings and photographs depicting dorsal fin shapes and body scars, they soon knew groups of non-provisioned dolphins, too. They found that the dolphins existed in fission–fusion groups or parties similar to those of chimpanzees; party members in one place at the same time were usually within two meters (6.5 ft) of each other or as much as ten meters (33 ft) apart; members of a party were never all together at any one time. The average number in a party was 4.8 adults, with a range of from two to 20 dolphins. Within parties were pairs or triplets of bonded males who often stayed together for years.

This bonding was most evident to the researchers when two males herded a female, who was presumably in estrus. A male would lure a female toward him by making a popping vocalization after which he and his fellow male, called partners, swam on either side of her, but slightly behind, so that she had difficulty escaping should she wish to do so. Often the males performed spectacular synchronous displays similar to those seen in captivity, perhaps to beguile the female? If the males were part of a triplet, the "odd-male-out" would switch frequently with one of the males partnering the female. These pairs or triplets were referred to as "first-order alliances" to distinguish them from "second-order alliances" formed by other dolphins trying to steal the female away from the former group – the researchers observed six of these disputes during their study. Sometimes alliances helped other alliances to obtain a female, but the researchers were unsure why this would happen. Would it be an example of nepotism? Of reciprocity? Of pseudo-reciprocity? There was no way of knowing, given the lack of information on the hereditary relationships of the individuals. Herding was certainly about sex, because although the researchers never saw an intromission, at various times they saw one or two males mount a herded female; sometimes both males, trying to mount from either side of the female, had an erection. The authors postulate that like the primate brain, brains of social marine species such as the dolphin are also greatly enlarged because of the vast amount of information he or she has to contain about scores of other individuals in order to cope with necessary social intricacies.

GREYLAG GEESE

We have discussed greylag geese (*Anser anser*), the birds beloved by Konrad Lorenz, as an example of a species that has long-term pair-bonds between breeding males and females. Pairs of male geese at Lorenz's sanctuary in Austria sometimes also became firmly bonded, although for a long time researchers did not know this because they could not tell males from females. Robert Huber and Michael Martys (1993) decided to analyze 16 years of behavioral data dealing with male pairs in a population of 130 tame, free-flying geese, for whom the sex of most individuals was known from inspection of their cloacas shortly after hatching. Each bird had colored leg rings so that it could be recognized from a distance. After the first male–male pairs in the Grünau flock were identified in 1975, these homosexual duos were found to represent a prominent social unit in their population, some liaisons persisting for 15 years. Sometimes two brothers bonded, in a few cases after their female partners had been lost. Less frequently, two unrelated ganders formed a close pair, indicating that familiarity between the males was probably involved in the pairings. Homosexual pairs, which tended to hang out at the periphery of the flock, increased when the number of males in the population exceeded 55 percent.

The two men compared the behavior of six established gander pairs and six heterosexual pairs. Over 100 hours of observation from September 1983 until the following April, approach or avoidance aggressive behaviors and vocal sounds relating to social bonding (such as the triumph ceremony and warnings of danger) occurred in all of the pairs of geese, although the homosexual pairs had especially high levels of both agonistic and friendly behaviors, which in some cases seemed to terrorize the neighbors. There was no evidence that one of the male pair behaved in a pseudo-female way. One gander sometimes tried to mount the other after giving a precopulatory display, but such attempts did not always work well. He might eventually mount another goose entirely or a nearby log, although his postcopulatory display was always directed at his true partner. To reproduce, a male with a male partner may mate with a female whose eggs they then incubate. The apparent lack of female–female bonds in the population probably relates to the male bias in numbers and perhaps less strong pair-bonding behavior in females than in males.

Huber and Martys suggest various reasons why there were so many male–male couples in the population:

(a)   the male pairs with their vigilant behavior spent considerable time at the periphery of the flock to serve as watch-dogs for the entire flock;

(b)   the aggression of male pairs was usually directed at single ganders, so their activity may force these loners out of the flock, giving it more stability;

(c)   a pair-bond may be a better strategy for a gander than remaining single, as loners have a higher rate of predation and reduced access to resources;

(d)   male-pairing may represent a "buffer system" for males in a flock where the sex ratio is strongly male-biased; it keeps them socially fit in case a breeding possibility opens up in the future.

GREATER RHEAS

Two male rheas stymied avian experts. In 1995, scientists Gustavo Fernández and Juan Reboreda published a paper called "Adjacent nesting and egg stealing between males of the Greater Rhea *Rhea americana*." In this species, adult males in Argentina at the beginning of the breeding season establish a dominance hierarchy among themselves. The alpha male monopolizes as many females as he can, from three to ten, to persuade them to lay eggs in his "nest" that he has fashioned in the ground. This depression is about 15 to 30 cm (6–12 in) deep and one to 1.5 meters (3–5 ft) in diameter. After they copulate, females begin to lay their eggs beside his nest every two or three days; the male rolls them into the depression as they are produced. After several weeks, the male has up to 50 eggs accumulated, which he begins to incubate while the females prance away, their work completed. The male remains at his job for about six weeks, with only a few minutes off each day to eat and drink. He is constantly alert to prevent predators or other rheas from approaching his nest, threatening them aggressively or even chasing them away if necessary. When the myriad of precocial young hatch, they constantly remain with him, feeding and moving about together until the next breeding season.

What puzzled the scientists was that on four occasions during their three-year study of 350 greater rheas with 138 nests, four pairs of males produced two nests less than a meter (3 ft) apart. The evidence indicated that one nest had been built some time before the second one, so presumably one male had courted the females and then, during incubation, a friendly male had decided to join him. The number of eggs in either type of nest was similar, with the common single nests averaging 26 eggs and these double nests 28 eggs. The two males sat on their nests comfortably side by side, without any sign of aggression. They even exchanged eggs, which the scientists had marked with waterproof ink for identification. If one male went off for a break, the other could still keep all the eggs protected. The hatching success of the double nests was about 80 percent, while that of the single nests 66 percent. The chicks from the double nest had two adult males to care for them while those from the single nest had only one, so likely more of the former group survived to adulthood than of the latter.

The authors cast this whole episode as an example of egg stealing, as the title of their paper indicates, and discuss the possible causes of this "bizarre," "misdirected" behavior and its possible evolutionary implications:

(a)   Perhaps the second male hung around the nest as a female was laying her first and second eggs, and thus had a chance to mate with her? Therefore, the chance of eggs with his DNA hatching would be increased.

(b)   Perhaps the second male, who has given his time and attention to the eggs and young he did not sire, acquires nesting experience or has a better hope of attracting attention from a female in the future? (The males themselves were not marked, so they could have been exchanging nests now and then.)

(c)   Perhaps the males were related, such as brothers, so that the second male would also have a genetic interest in the chicks?

(d)   Perhaps the two males shared and mated with the same group of females so that both had good reason to rear the chicks? The researchers had, on occasion, seen "harems" with two males.

The answer to this conundrum seems to me to be friendship. If a male has his own clutch of eggs destroyed by a predator or other catastrophe, he might decide to join a buddy as he is already, physiologically, in a care-giving mood. On the other hand, he may not have attracted any females at all, but still be willing to help a pal in raising his young (as he himself has no hope of breeding until the next season); or he may not be interested in breeding. (There are reports of homosexual behavior, often quite common, in all the related species of rhea, emu, ostrich, and cassowary [Bagemihl, 1999].) The eggs were not stolen, but shifted over from one nest to the other where they would have received equal attention – males are already programmed to shift nearby eggs laid by a female into their nest. In addition, this double-nest friendship has the potential to be more successful than usual in raising chicks because there are two caring males rather than one to do the job.

BLACK SWANS

Black swans have been of interest to philosophers of science ever since Karl Popper used them as an example of an alternative scientific method based on falsification. For centuries, Europeans were familiar with the swans that inhabited their countries. Because all of them were white, they assumed that all swans were white. They could not prove this, however, no matter how many white swans they saw. Popper proposed that it would be better not to keep adding more evidence of white swans, but to try to disprove the hypothesis. This occurred when Europeans visited Australia for the first time and saw black swans. Even a single black swan would repudiate the hypothesis that all swans were white.

The black swans (*Cygnus atratus*) of Australia and New Zealand have other surprises too. Some males form strong bonds of affection with each other, staying together for years (Bagemihl, 1999). They often perform the greeting ceremony to cement and reinforce their partnership; this involves the two birds facing each other, raising their wings, extending their necks and bills toward the sky, and calling repeatedly. Another behavior common also to heterosexual pairs is head-dipping, a prelude to copulation. The pair of swans immerse first their heads, then their necks, and finally their whole bodies in water in a wave-like fashion, a display that can continue for 20 minutes or more and may or may not lead to one male mounting the other.

In order to raise young, the pair obtain fertile eggs in a nest in one of two ways: either they associate with a female, building a nest together and mating with her, then chasing her away when her eggs are laid, or both males take over a nest with eggs from a heterosexual couple by force. They take turns sitting on and incubating the eggs and, when the young are hatched, look after them as they grow. Two males are especially effective in raising cygnets because, together, they are larger and stronger than a usual couple and able to defend, for themselves, a territory far bigger than that of most pairs. On average, 80 percent of young are raised successfully by two fathers, while the success rate for heterosexual parents is only about 30 percent. In any one year, about 13 percent of black swans are involved in homosexual pair-bonds, a percentage that in some cases rises to 20 percent.

Mute swans (*Cygnus olor*) may form female as well as male homosexual pair-bonds, but the eggs that the female couples lay are infertile and do not hatch. Nevertheless, the swans stay together, presumably valuing their friendship more than the possibility of producing and rearing young.

HUMBOLDT PENGUINS

Male Humboldt or Peruvian penguin pairs (*Spheniscus humboldti*) sometimes form lifelong friendships that last as long as six years, until one of them dies (Bagemihl, 1999). When they are not at sea hunting for fish, like heterosexual pairs they spend much of their time close together, often in contact, either in an underground burrow they have built or in a rough niche above ground. They may give the ecstatic display, which involves males, either alone or standing beside their partner, stretching their head and neck up, spreading their flippers wide, and flapping them while giving several long calls that sound like the loud braying of a donkey. The pair may also bow to each other and allogroom, running their bills through their partner's sleek feathers. Prior to copulation, one male approaches the other from behind, pressing his body against that of his partner, and vibrating his flippers. For mounting, one male lies down on his stomach and holds his tail to the side while the other climbs onto his back so that their cloacas can touch. Then they may reverse positions. The homosexual pairs do not try to raise young, however, and seem content with their close friendship. As well as such permanent homosexual pairs, other males may be bisexual in behavior or choose to mate with a male who is part of a heterosexual couple.

LONG-TAILED MANAKINS

Seldom is the social system of a species dominated by culture, especially a culture based on partnerships, but this is the case for the long-tailed manakin (*Chiroxiphia linearis*). These birds, sometimes called fandango birds because of the males' wild gyrations (the word taken from lively dances of Spanish or African origin), live high in the mountains of Costa Rica. The black males are secretive but striking, with scarlet caps, sky blue backs, long tail feathers, and glorious vocalizations.

They live in male groups of up to 15 birds with a linear dominance hierarchy. During the courtship season, they gather at a perch zone, also known as a lek or display ground, where primarily the duo alpha and beta birds perform amazing song duets and dance routines to impress the females, who come by themselves or in a small group to check out the presentations and to mate with the alpha male if they like what they hear and see. The duet, which attracts females to the singers' perch zone from long distances away, is a short melody sung by one bird and repeated a fraction of a second later by the second bird. If a team of two males has well-matched voices, their perch zone is especially attractive to females. As soon as a female arrives, the alpha and beta males (usually) begin their courtship performance involving the joint backwards leapfrog dance. This goes on for one or several lengthy bouts until the female leaves or agrees to mate.

Male manakins visit various groups of males as they grow, interacting with different partners in each group. By the age of four years, they have reached their final, bright-colored, mature plumage, and a few years after this, have narrowed down their preferred partners. Birds aged seven years with beta status usually interact at only two perch zones, while alpha birds of perhaps ten years almost always perform with their beta chum at only one perch zone site. Alpha–beta partnerships take years to consolidate, gradually becoming more stable as older males display with fewer and fewer partners. The following authors note that their "network of social interactions is arguably as complex as that found in any non-human society," but eventually an alpha and beta hook up as one talented singing and dancing team.

The alpha and beta males are not usually related, so why is the beta bird willing to wait for up to ten years to mate with females, when he may become the alpha male himself? This was the question that intrigued the research team of Jill Trainer, David McDonald, and William Learn (2002), who studied the birds by identifying individuals by color bands and plumage, and tape-recording the singing repertoires of various pairs and the repercussions these had on females. Singing competence increased as the beta bird grew older and, with practice, frequency matching by established teams also improved. The researchers conclude that the beta bird remains a stable partner rather than a rival of the alpha bird for mating opportunities, for four reasons:

(a)   he may eventually become an alpha male himself;
(b)   he may, on rare occasions, mate with females if the alpha bird is temporarily absent;

(c)   the females usually remain faithful to a particular perch zone even with a change in alpha birds;

(d)   beta birds gradually increase their competence at displays, which helps to attract more females for the older alpha males. Because well-performed songs attract more females to a perch zone and stimulate females to mate, a beta male, with his improved singing, should eventually have good mating success should he himself inherit the perch zone along with the females who are faithful to this site. Only about eight percent of first-year manakin males will ever become alpha birds with the potential to copulate, so working in tandem with their partners at perfecting their singing and dancing has at last paid off in spades for successful beta manakins.

In summary, close friendships between males offer various kinds of advantages within many species: companionship, allogrooming, joint leadership, coalitions within a group or to fight other groups, sex, sharing of meat, lending of status from a dominant to a subordinate animal, increased mating opportunities, and rarely raising young together.

For an infant daughter, her mother is her whole world. As we shall see in the following chapter, her attachment lessens as she grows into maturity but, especially for monkeys, it often remains firm in her adulthood. This friendship that involves such communal activities as feeding, resting, traveling, allogrooming, and keeping a watch out for danger benefits both mother and daughter.

Mothers and daughters

In all mammals, the bond between mother and daughter is tight at birth, with the infant staying close to her parent for support and comfort as well as for milk. As the youngster grows, however, she becomes increasingly independent. This shift has been documented for Soay sheep living on the Scottish island of St. Kilda (Clutton-Brock *et al.*, 2004). They are free-ranging and thought to be intermediate in type between wild sheep and domestic sheep; the latter have had their social instincts bred out of them to some extent so that they will perceive a shepherd as their leader rather than an elderly ewe (Darling, 1969). Although they seldom interact with their mother, Soay juvenile and yearling daughters usually graze within 20 meters (22 yd) of her as their mutual bond weakens (Clutton-Brock *et al.*, 2004). (The bond between mother and son dissolves much faster, with the lamb on his own by six months of age.) By the time the daughter is about two years old, this friendship is gone, too. She is no more likely to associate with her mother than with any other female in their group. From a human point of view, it is nice to know that the mother likely will, by that time, have another young offspring at heel.

In other species such as those described as follows (chimpanzees, gorillas, baboons, Japanese monkeys, and ring-tailed lemurs), some daughters remain close to their mothers when they reach maturity, continuing to interact with her in a variety of ways. These species are all primates. Presumably other species have close mother–adult daughter ties, too, but research has not focused on this possibility.

FLO AND FIFI, CHIMPANZEES

Flo was the first animal to become famous worldwide because of Jane Goodall's research. She was a wonderful mother to Fifi, her only

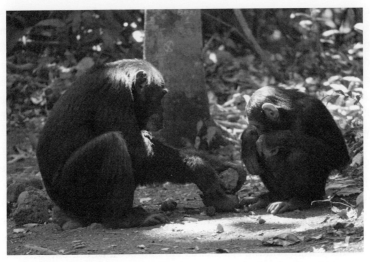

Figure 4. A mother cracks oil palm nuts, watched by her daughter.
© Susana Carvalho

daughter to reach adulthood. Flo was about 32 years of age when Goodall first saw her in 1961. When, in 1962, she came to the feeding area near the camp that Goodall had set up, she was accompanied by Fifi, then a youngster, and her juvenile son Figan (Goodall, 1986). The following year when she was in estrus, Flo was followed by a number of randy males, in this way introducing them to the free bananas at the feeding station that they had not realized existed.

Throughout her life, Fifi had a tight social bond with Flo, who was aggressive and highly ranked, but also an affectionate, tolerant, and playful mother; indeed, Flo would be the only female with whom Fifi formed a close friendship. Flo played with Fifi and her other youngsters by grabbing at their feet as they chased around a tree, or tickling and mock biting them. When Flo groomed another chimpanzee, Fifi often slipped between the two so that her mother would groom her instead. Several times when they were fishing for termites with sticks, Fifi came whimpering to Flo because the hole she was working with no longer yielded the insects. Flo courteously (unlike other mothers) let her use her more productive hole and went herself to find another. Fifi, who chose not to emigrate when she reached puberty, was always supported and protected by Flo when she was involved in conflicts. When Fifi was in late adolescence, she travelled with males during her sexual swelling, but she always returned to be with her mother after her swelling subsided. Neither female liked to see the other copulating with a male, so each would rush forward to try to stop this activity.[1] (Foreshadowing of similar perspectives between human mothers and daughters?) After her son Freud was born in 1971, Fifi continued to hang out with Flo, the two fond grooming partners. Their close bond was only loosened in the last few months of Flo's life, when she was too frail and old to travel. She remained in a tiny area in the Kasakela Valley where, presumably, there was not enough food for Fifi, who now had little Freud to care for.

Fifi had a fine legacy because of Flo's friendship and influence. She became an excellent mother, as Flo had been, spending large amounts of time feeding and resting with her growing family, which would eventually comprise two sons and two daughters (Goodall, 1986). Fifi was often aggressive in her relationships with other females, so frequently displaying and attacking them that she became a high-ranking female, as Flo had been before her. She was extremely attractive to males when she was in estrus, calmly crouching down so that they could mount her as Flo had done, perhaps in part because she had grown up with two brothers and was used to male company. Like Flo, she was also fond of meat. As an infant and juvenile, she had watched many meat-eating sessions of chimpanzees where Flo was experienced and persistent in cadging portions of monkey, bushpig, or bushbuck flesh from those who had caught these animals. Sometimes, when frustrated male bystanders attacked her for her persistence, she ran away screaming, but she was soon back to continue begging. Several years before she died, Flo attended two such sessions in which she managed to scrounge two large chunks of meat for herself. After Flo's death, Fifi took part in many hunting parties that caught a number of medium-sized animals; two weeks after giving birth, she herself raced 200 meters (220 yd) after a mother–infant pair of colobus monkeys, supporting her own tiny infant with one hand, to nab the mother and then the baby. She and her son, who was trying to keep up with her, then ate both of them. Flo would have been proud.

PASSION AND POM, CHIMPANZEES

Pom was born to Passion (then of unknown age) in 1965. She proved to be a very bad mother, rearing her youngster, as described by Jane Goodall (1986), with "extraordinarily inefficient and indifferent maternal behavior." When Pom cried because she was hungry, Passion did not guide the infant's mouth to her nipple, but made Pom find it for herself. When Pom grew older, Passion did not always gather her up in her arms to tuck her under her body when she moved away, but might simply walk on, leaving Pom to scamper after her, whimpering (Montgomery, 1991).

Pom and Passion as adults would share a tight social bond and a rare one – that of being cooperative baby killers, biting infants in the forehead, and cannibals who then ate the small bodies. Passion, in 1975, was able to stalk and snatch Gilka's infant, but Gilka was small and weak at the time; her arm and hand were partly paralysed from a polio epidemic (Goodall, 1986). The following year, when she had produced another infant, Gilka was able to put up a stronger fight against Passion. She might have saved her baby had not Pom joined the attack. During this assault and another on Melissa's infant, Passion and Pom worked together as a coordinated team. The heavier and stronger Passion struggled with the mother while Pom pulled at the baby. They were not antagonistic toward Melissa once they had her baby; in the one case when Melissa approached Passion and Pom as they were eating her infant, Passion reached out to embrace her and the two mothers briefly held hands. In 1978, Passion had a long and violent battle with Miff during which the two fell six meters (20 ft) to the ground, but she was unable to grab Miff's infant without Pom's help; Pom was pregnant at the time and did not join in the attack. Passion may have been unsuccessful in part because she was hindered by her four-month-old infant. When Pom joined in the attack so that they worked together, they were observed over a four-year period to grab, kill, and eat three tiny infants and may have taken as many as seven others. (Adult males were also seen to attack and kill chimpanzee infants, but these had all belonged to mothers from other communities.) Both Passion and Pom were high ranking, which was uncommon for female dyads, a status surely related to the fear they aroused in other females because of their infanticide.

Passion and Pom were jointly involved in eating the meat of other species, too, which provided an additional source of protein. On two occasions in 1977, they devoured a newborn bushbuck fawn which Passion had caught, killed, and shared with her new infant and with Pom. Passion consumed the brains and an ear (along with leaves) while Pom drank blood from the mouth and ears, and then munched on the hooves and viscera. The family ate slowly, taking almost five hours to reduce their prey to a tangle of skin, leg bones, and spine. Pom occasionally took part in group hunts with males, but from these she obtained less meat than when she joined her family in their own hunting unit. Passion usually did not hunt other species, although she was willing to eat some meat (never a great deal) from fawns and piglets when this was available from group hunts. Probably the dyad's success in obtaining protein strengthened their bond of friendship.

As she grew older, Passion spent almost all her time with family, which included Pom, Passion's two sons born after Pom, and Pom's infant born in 1978. In 1977, Passion had travelled more extensively than usual in order to accompany Pom who was in estrus and moving about with adult males. Both females were tense and excitable (unlike Flo and Fifi) when mating. When Pom's youngster died at the age of three years in 1981, the bond between mother and daughter became stronger than ever. They were almost always together during Passion's final illness from a wasting disease. She died in 1982. Pom and the older brother cared for Passion's last born, little Pax, but Pom herself was no longer seen after late 1983.

GRAY AND ZIRA, CHIMPANZEES

Michael Ghiglieri (1988) does not know without doubt that Gray and Zira were mother and daughter because his field-work in the Kibale Forest of Uganda lasted for only two years, but they were such close friends that he assumed this must be so. Female chimpanzees in general do not form friendships with non-relatives. Gray, an old wrinkled female, and Zira, a sleek young adult, spent much of their time together, and were closer than any other two adults he observed during his research (although a few other chimpanzees also had preferred friends of the same sex). Zira was more skittish, however. At first, as he sat with binoculars watching chimpanzees feed in a fig tree, Ghiglieri noticed that every time he shifted position, even though he was quite far away, Zira would panic and rush down an exit tree. But soon she would be back, having realized that Gray and the other chimpanzees were still calmly stuffing their faces. Gradually, she became used to his presence. However, on one occasion he climbed into a tree to escape from a herd of elephants milling below; he sat perched there for an hour after they had moved on, thinking about the good view and the security a tree offered (although it came with more mosquitoes than on the ground). When Gray and Zira chanced to glance up as they were passing below him, however, they bolted.

A man sitting at a distance staring up at them was one thing, but that man hanging out in a tree, their domain, was something else again.

Gray and Zira each loved to be groomed, which involved one grooming the other who then would reciprocate, a mutual activity which completely engrossed them. Indeed, they held the record in Ghiglieri's field notes for having the longest session of mutual grooming – two hours and three minutes, with some time off for self-grooming or staring into space; Gray groomed Zira 20 times for a total of 52 minutes and Zira reciprocated 19 times for a total of 49 minutes. During such sessions they had ample time to inspect most parts of each other's bodies at least once. Social grooming was important for all the chimpanzees at Ngogo, especially after foraging when tensions were at their lowest. Being groomed was better than grooming, so there was friendly competition to try and prolong being a groomee rather than a groomer. Usually the individual being groomed presented one body part after another that needed attention until the groomer had had enough, when their positions were reversed. Ghiglieri was amazed by the friendship, reassurance, and unqualified trust exhibited between two grooming partners whose individual space and usual protocols were completely suppressed.

MOUNTAIN GORILLAS

Mountain gorilla female duos are not known for their close friend-ships, because in this species as in hamadryas baboons and chim-panzees, it is the adolescent female who usually departs from her natal troop and joins another, leaving her mother and other friends behind. Female gorilla and chimpanzee duos do become close friends sometimes, though, as we saw in the chapter: In sisterhood.

Alexander Harcourt (1979) decided to observe close female friendships in gorillas by observing and recording, over a two-year period, the behavior of some of the same animals Dian Fossey knew.[2] Gorillas were difficult to watch because Harcourt often had to tramp a long way from camp to where various groups were hanging out, and then the members were not always visible in dense vegetation; around midday was the best time to see them when they were resting rather than foraging or traveling. Nevertheless, he carried on and discovered that, actually, a mother and her daughter who had remained in the troop *were* special buddies (in Dian Fossey's group 5), as were another pair of females (in group 4) who had grown up together from immaturity. All the other females in these troops merely tolerated each other – if two were seen together, it was usually because they both wanted to be close to the silverback male who headed the group. Harcourt used check sheets divided into columns for behavior and rows for time intervals. On them, he noted when two animals were close together (within two or five meters [about 6.5 or 16 ft]), touching, or grooming. Where possible, he also recorded who of a pair initiated an activity and who ended it; a "positive responsibility index" noted which individual was more responsible for the activity.

The mother–daughter team and the long-term dyad observed by Harcourt did spend more time together than did other females, and it was the daughter of the first duo who was the more responsible for maintaining this proximity. Both pairs liked touching each other, the mother and daughter especially, sometimes sitting or lying together for minutes. Both pairs groomed more than did other females, with the younger partner the more active; the daughter was particularly assiduous in grooming her mother who rarely reciprocated. Harcourt generalizes that for primates there are two main reasons for adopting friendly behavior toward other individuals, both of which are selfish. One is that friendly interactions should be directed toward animals more *likely* to help them if needed, which includes relatives and those close in the hierarchical ranking. The second is that they should be addressed toward individuals who are more *able* to help, which includes higher-ranking and more experienced individuals.

Harcourt muses about why females might be willing to allow non-relatives to join their troop, as this could reduce the amount of food available and perhaps increase aggression. He suggests four reasons:

(a)   the leading male could prevent the smaller adult females from expelling immigrating females;
(b)   food is usually abundant rather than limited;
(c)   more troop members might increase feeding efficiency by a coordination of travel routes and the consequent maintenance of quality forage;
(d)   more females would mean more infants available to play with the infants of the original females.

SYLVIA AND SIERRA, CHACMA BABOONS

Sylvia (born in 1982) and her eldest daughter Sierra (born in 1989) lived in Botswana's Okavango Delta where Anne Engh and her colleagues (2006) and Dorothy Cheney and Robert Seyfarth (2007) all spent many years observing and interacting with the approximately 80 members of Troop C, which were chacma baboons (*Papio hamadryas ursinus*). Old Sylvia was called by the researchers the "Queen of Mean" because she was high-ranking, aggressive, and took no nonsense from anybody. When she moved through her troop, cantankerous and irritable, lesser females and juveniles scattered before her. If some did not get out of her way fast enough, she bit or whacked them (Cheney and Seyfarth, 2007).

As her daughter, Sierra also ranked high in the female dominance hierarchy. Cheney and Seyfarth give two examples of how relationships in the hierarchy worked. When Sierra was a juvenile, she was walking one day toward a jackalberry tree where other baboons were feeding. The low-ranking Jeanette who was in her path did not move aside as she should have done following baboon protocol, but instead gave a head bob threat. Sierra immediately lunged at her in retaliation for her presumption, giving a series of threat-grunts and a scream. Her actions not only threatened Jeanette, but broadcast her anger to her female relatives. Sylvia and two aunts rushed to Sierra's aid, although actually Sierra was in no trouble at all. All four jumped on Jeanette, pinning her to the ground and biting her tail. Jeanette dropped the food she had been eating, wrestled free, and fled screaming, but no one responded to her calls as relatives had to those of Sierra. Only high-ranking maternal relatives look after their own.

On another occasion, Sierra approached Hannah, a new mother and seventh-ranked female who had been prevented from eating or resting all morning because higher-ranking females had been crowding in to inspect and handle her infant. When Sierra came by to do the same thing, it was apparently the last straw for Hannah. She grabbed Sierra's hand and slapped her face. This action again violated baboon protocol, but Sierra did not retaliate immediately as she might have. Nevertheless, she remembered the incident. An hour later, she again approached Hannah who drew back reflexively, but relaxed when Sierra grunted in apparent friendship. When Sierra reached her, however, she leapt on her and bit her neck.

Sylvia and Sierra were an important part of experiments carried out by Cheney and Seyfarth, who wanted to know how each baboon living in the troop perceived his or her troop-mates. To do this, over many months they collected an archive of calls emitted by known individuals. From these, they could select a specific call to be sent out over a loudspeaker and observe how baboons within ear range reacted. The researchers discovered, by using such play-back recordings of individuals giving a variety of calls, that all the baboons in the troop recognized Sylvia's distinctive voice (and undoubtedly the voice of other individuals as well), no matter if she were giving a grunt, a contact bark, or a threat-grunt, and doing so loudly or softly, or in a calm or agitated manner. A baboon such as Sylvia would ignore a sequence such as "Sierra threat-grunts and Luxe [another baboon] screams," but would respond strongly to "Luxe threat-grunts and Sierra screams."

Sylvia had six other offspring and Sierra five young, but it was to each other that they were especially devoted. They were tight friends, greeting each other with lipsmacks, a universal sign of friendly intentions in all monkeys, and with amiable grunts common in baboon language. They spent a great deal of time grooming each other, which reinforced their bond. But then a lion killed Sierra when Sylvia was 21, and her grief at the loss of her best friend and grooming partner was great. She fell into what could only be described as a depression. The level of glucocorticoids in her blood increased – stress levels in a baboon rise with the death of a grooming partner or close relative as well as when their own social ranking is in danger, both risk factors for old Sylvia.

The researchers had hypothesized that with her main grooming partner gone, a female such as Sylvia would have fewer baboons with whom to interact and groom. In fact, what happened was the opposite. At first Sylvia's stress hormones increased, but by the second month after the death, her glucocorticoid levels returned to baseline. With this change, Sylvia was largely able to slough off her depression from Sierra's death. Her need for social contact was so great that she deigned to down-play her superiority and embarked on a grooming campaign. She began to approach other females, startling them by grunting a greeting and attempting to groom them. Her particular focus was Atchar, a low-ranking female who was at first terrified of Sylvia because of her bad reputation. She fled in a panic when Sylvia approached her with raspy grunts. Gradually, however, Sylvia gained new friends and enough grooming mates to be able to carry on more or less contentedly in her troop, despite the loss of her daughter and best friend.

JAPANESE MONKEYS

Like baboons, Japanese monkeys live in large multimale and multi-female groups. As we saw in the chapter: *In sisterhood*, Masayuki Nakamichi and K. Yamada (2007) analyzed friendships among 18 free-ranging adult females in Japan that had lasted for ten years, between 1993 and 2003. The hereditary maternal relationships of the monkeys were known for a number of generations. Friendship was measured by grooming bouts carried out between two animals, affiliative behavior considered important in establishing and maintaining social bonds. Data were collected during the two daily provisioning sessions when monkeys tended to stay in clusters in the open feeding area and where any grooming between two female pairs could easily be recorded by a person on foot. From these results, grooming between dyads who were related and those who were not was compared.

In general, grooming is kin-based in Japanese monkey females, occurring most often between mothers and their adult daughters (but also between sisters), cementing a long-term psychological bond. Mother–daughter bonds are continuous and strong until one of the dyad disappears from the troop, usually because of death. There is a dominance hierarchy in the species whereby the mother is dominant to her daughters and a younger sister is dominant to an older one. Because of this, the frequency of grooming between mother and an older daughter tends to decrease over time, while that between the mother and younger daughter(s) increases. (Having a newborn sister routinely become dominant over her older sister is a difficult concept to grasp. It is similar to a man marrying a second wife, whereupon she often becomes dominant over the first wife, in part because the husband gives her more attention, just as the mother monkey gives her youngest infant the most attention. What a nightmare sibling rivalry would be if this openly pertained to human beings! What a godsend for psychiatrists!)

RING-TAILED LEMURS

Ring-tailed lemurs (*Lemur catta*) fight more than other primates (Sussman and Garber, 2004) but mothers and grown daughters, or sister pairs, may form fast friendships. Female adults have little time for males, who are all subordinate to them. They come into estrus at about the same time each year, but only for a one-day period during which each chooses the males with whom she will copulate. Over as short a period as one week, all adult males of a troop compete fiercely among themselves in the hope of attracting female attention.

Masayuki Nakamichi from Osaka University, Japan, an inveterate observer of various primate species for his research, set out with his colleague Naoki Koyama (1997) to study the social relationships of ring-tailed lemurs living in two free-ranging troops in Madagascar. These animals were used to human voyeurs, so it was easy for the researchers to see and note down what individuals were doing and with whom they hung out every day, over a three-month period. They worked for three hours each morning and three hours each evening, when the lemurs were most active. At first light, the drill began by choosing at random the first lemur to be the focal animal of the 32 individuals, half in each troop. Each focal animal was observed for ten minutes before going on to the next (or the animal after that, if the target one could not be located during the next ten minutes). Animals closer than two meters (6.5 ft) to the target lemur were noted, as was the absence of any lemur within five meters (16 ft), indicating that she or he was alone. Grooming using the tooth-comb (lower incisors and canines modified by evolution for this purpose) was recorded, along with timing the animal that was doing the grooming, or if they were grooming each other at the same time. In addition, the researchers noted down any excitements or unusual activities such as dominance or submission interactions or battles with neighboring troops. At the close of the study, they had 12 hours of observational data for each lemur, along with 186 hours of notes about other events that had occurred during the three months.

The results confirmed that some female pairs in the troops liked to be with each other. Four of these were mother–adult daughter duos who spent 30 to 40 percent of their time close together, and groomed each other much more often than other individuals. They were also more active in defending their feeding grounds at territorial boundaries by fighting for their own troop against others, slashing out with their razor-sharp upper canines. However, these females were not involved much in coalitions: 53 percent of aggressive interactions involved only one female from either group battling, with neither supported by a colleague. Because one female was usually left to fight an enemy by herself, daughters did not benefit from the dominance ranking of their mothers, as happens in many primate species. Although the females did most of the fighting, they were not much bothered by strange solitary males who wandered into their territory; these were attacked largely by the males instead, who did not want more rivals around to eat the group's food or mate with the females.

But these facts and figures do not give a flavor of the mother–daughter soap opera that is a staple of ring-tailed lemur life. In her book *Lords and Lemurs*, Alison Jolly (2004), who studied the species in southern Madagascar for over fifty years, details the trials and tribulations of members of the A-team of Berenty. Diva was the A-team's original alpha animal, a female so ensconced in power that none in her troop dared cross her or her daughter, the "delicate beauty" Jessica who clung to her mother's side. Diva did not have to chase or chastise other group members because they all kept out of her way. Fish was the third-ranked female of the A-team in 1990, the year her daughter Fan was born. Both mothers were best friends with their grown daughters, the two resting together and often grooming each other's soft fur. Fish was an aggressive animal, subservient to Diva but active in badgering lemurs ranked below her in the troop hierarchy. By the time Fan was two years old, full size although not yet a mother, she worked with Fish to harass the more subordinate animals. They finally managed to oust this lowly group from the troop in 1992, when there was a drought that reduced the available food supply. Such ousting was a terrible fate, leaving the outcasts with no territory of their own where they could feed. They had to slink about without being detected, hoping to slip into food trees claimed by rival troops.

This outcast group of low-ranking lemurs, now named the Exiles, included young mothers called Shadow and Sly. While Jolly watched, Shadow gave birth to her first child during one of their routs after moving slightly away from the other resting, exhausted Exile members. She had half an hour to lick her newborn before she had to move on with the group – it was essential to stay together for fear of predators or of other ringtails. Sly's infant would be lost in combat, as would that of Blotch, another Exile female.

But then came a battle for existence and an innovation in behavior that Jolly had never seen before. Usually in troop confrontations, one animal from each side came forward to fight. The rest watched. This time Sly, Shadow, and the three other females presented a united front to the enemy, Fish and Fan. The five leapt onto the roof of a bungalow and glared down as a cohesive group at the fierce mother–daughter pair. Shadow was the first to launch herself at the duo who immediately backed off, fearing to turn around lest they be jumped on from behind. It was an historic moment for the Exiles, soon to be renamed the Together group. They immediately swarmed into a eucalyptus grove belonging to the A-team to stuff themselves full of buds and flowers. "The new troop had earned their reward. All around them the air

smelled of honey," Jolly writes. Quickly victory followed victory, eucalyptus tree after eucalyptus tree was occupied, until the Together group,
with its new confidence and fighting style, had regained the best of the
former A-team territory. Once they were sure that this new group would
survive, four males joined it permanently. Shadow's infant was the only
youngster to survive the turmoil, but because he was a son rather than a
daughter, he would not grow up to be Shadow's best friend or to help her
group thrive.

What of Diva and Jessica, and Fish and Fan of the A-team? The
mother–daughter duos were now cast down. They had made a huge
mistake by driving away the subordinates in their group. The advances
the Together troop made into the original A-team territory meant that
there was only a small piece of inferior real estate left for them. Diva
plummeted from power, spending her final two years skulking about at
the periphery of the troop. Without her mother's protection, her daughter Jessica fell too, remaining at the bottom of the hierarchy after her
mother's death. She became thin and stringy instead of lithe, her fur
molting in patches on her thighs. Fish took over as alpha female, to be
succeeded by her daughter Fan, but there was little glory in the position
now that the troop had lost so much. Frightful Fan, as Jolly called her,
became increasingly angry, perhaps in part because she kept producing
sons instead of daughters, which undercut her ambition for more power.
In 1997 she drove Jessica, her niece, and their infants out of her troop
entirely. There was barely enough food to go around, so whenever Fan
saw Jessica, she chased her away at top speed for hundreds of meters.
When the A-team had split up in 1992, the inferior portion had tri-
umphed, but that did not happen again. Jessica and her children never
gained a territory of their own; the members gradually disappeared or
died until finally there was no one left of haughty Diva's lineage.

In summary, mothers are important and may be best friends to
their daughters. Their joint activities include allogrooming, sharing
meat, forming aggressive coalitions, and mothers "teaching" daughters by their example, giving them higher status, and helping them in
times of distress.

Most sons, as adults, do not live in the same group as their
mothers, but when they do, the mother can be a big help to them, as
we shall see in the next chapter. If she has a dominant personality, she
can act as back-up so that any males challenging him will have to take
on his mother, too. If animals belong to a solitary species, a mother and
son may still join together to hunt.

Mothers and sons, and providing free food

Social females rarely live in groups with their adult sons, presumably, according to evolutionary theory, to avoid inbreeding. If a son does stay with his natal group when he reaches maturity, he might mate with his mother, as has been seen rarely for chimpanzees (Goodall, 1986). For example, in a small family of gibbons in Thailand (*Hylobates lar*), the adult male disappeared leaving his presumed son, almost an adult at eight years of age, with his mother and an empty territory (Brockelman *et al.*, 1998). The son duetted with his mother and could have set up a new life with her, but instead chose to leave both her and their domain.

When mothers and adult sons do live in the same group, however, and if she is high-ranking in a species with a dominance hierarchy, she can be of great help to her son. It is to her advantage to help increase the chances that he will become a breeding male who can pass along their DNA to the next generation. Here we will consider the behaviors of bonobos, chimpanzees, woolly spider monkeys, coyotes, leopards, and lastly, the pros and cons of researchers providing food such as bananas and sugar cane to "their" animals. This activity has both positive (it speeds up individual identification and habituation of the animals) and negative (it interferes with the natural lives of the animals and fosters unnatural behavior to an unknown extent) results.

BONOBOS

A mother's adult daughters will usually each produce a number of youngsters in her lifetime and in this way carry on the inheritance her mother has bequeathed her. By contrast, her adult sons, if they belong to a polygamous species, may sire a large number of offspring or none at all. It makes genetic sense, therefore, for a mother to help her son where possible to function as a breeding male. As we have seen, bonobos are very sociable animals; both female friends and heterosexual couples may form close bonds, and so may mothers and their sons. Indeed, blood may trump a female's other friendships, with the bonobo, the poster species for mother–son bonding.

When young bonobos are growing up, they go everywhere with their mother, clinging to her fur, riding on her back, or following along behind her. When the young females reach adolescence, well before they are ready to reproduce they become less social, losing interest in their family ties (Kano, 1992). They hang around by themselves at the edge of the group for a while and then suddenly depart, transferring to another troop entirely. The mother–daughter bond is completely extinguished and there will be no possibility of inbreeding between the young female and the local males, one of whom is likely her father.

By contrast, young males continue to stay with their mother. The mother–son bond is formed during the son's earliest years, when bonobos develop more slowly than do young chimpanzees. Mothers are very attentive to their young during this time, sharing intense communication with them (de Waal, 1997), and this closeness between mother and son remains strong throughout their lives. Early on, because females are dominant to males, this bond may be a necessity because other females can drive all males out of a fruiting tree; sometimes, only when a mother and son are alone are they able to feed in peace. Zoologists in the past, who have seen a male and female traveling together through the forest, have assumed they were a mated couple. However, they were really mother and son with no sexual interest in each other. Such a dyad travels from one source of food to another along with other bonobos in a larger group or unit with ever-changing members. The son gains rank from his mother's dominance while his mother benefits from her son's presence as protector for her younger infants (Hohmann et al., 1999).

During adolescence and early adulthood, a son spends more time grooming with his mother than with anyone else and almost always forages with her. Such pairs visited provisioning centers such as that organized at Wamba, Zambia, by Takayoshi Kano (1992). Relationships between mothers and sons could be monitored by recording the presence of both at the same time at a feeding station and the distance between them (Ihobe, 1992). When an older female approached the sugar cane piles set out for the bonobos, low-ranking males quickly got out of her way, while the higher-ranking ones turned their backs to protect their food morsels or fled on two legs, clutching the food to their chests. Sometimes a son would beg for food from his mother and receive it, but the reverse situation was extremely rare. (Bonobos, although more gregarious than chimpanzees, are less likely to share food with each other, probably because their sources of quality food are larger and more available than are those of chimpanzees [Kano, 1992].)

Sons may be problematic for mothers at times. A bonobo mother will counter an attack on her adolescent or adult son, but he is seldom seen to return the favor, although this may be because middle-aged females are seldom assaulted. Kano describes one such rare event. A young adult male called Ten attacked and bit an old female, Kame. He held her down while she screamed, attracting her son Mon, who had been feeding 20 meters (65 feet) away. Mon leapt to her defence as did her older son Ibo; Ten's mother Sen also jumped into the fray on behalf of her own son, and the assault ended in a flurry of black fur.

If a mother is raising two male youngsters, one an infant and the other about five years old, these males are, in general, tolerant of each other, but two or three older sons do not form a powerful alliance as they might were they chimpanzees. As adults, bonobo sons are fortunate if they have a high-ranking mother because their own dominance in the male hierarchy depends largely on her presence rather than on the sons allying themselves with other males. As de Waal (2005) notes, "Instead of forming ever-changing coalitions among themselves, male bonobos vie for positions on their mothers' apron strings."

When the son is in a confrontation as an adult, the attacker knows that his dominant mother, his best friend, will back her son up. If the mother dies, however, his rank soon slips (de Waal, 1997). For example, Kame's eldest son, Ibo, was the alpha male of his group. Ten, the son of Sen, was the beta male. When Kame became too old and weak (and less popular sexually with both males and females because she no longer had her usual large swelling), Ten began to challenge her son, once defeating Ibo one-on-one in a fierce battle. However, the most critical conflict occurred not among the sturdy males but between the two mothers, in which Sen finally managed to vanquish Kame and hold her down as they rolled about on the ground. They had many skirmishes after this, but Kame never regained her dominance. As a result of Kame's defeat, Ibo lost his rank as alpha male to Ten. Kame's sons were ranked middle in the male hierarchy for several years until she died, when their dominance fell even farther. This plummet must be upsetting to the males, but it shows that having one's ranking dependent on another can give a false picture of one's abilities.

Bonobos have two unusual features in their social behavior: the mother–son bond is very strong and females are the dominant sex, even though they are slightly smaller than males. Are these facts related? Chimpanzees are much less likely to bond with their adult sons (with a few exceptions described in the following section), and dominance is very important in how a society functions. Frans de Waal (1997) hypothesizes that during the social evolution of bonobos, females began to have more frequent sexual swellings that lasted for longer, so that the number of sexual couplings increased, muting possible aggression. Males would often mate with females, and with more intense sexual activity, females began to have sex with females too, as did males with males to a lesser extent. De Waal notes that with females receptive much longer than in most communities (and certainly than in chimpanzee groups), there will be less fighting by males for the opportunity to copulate. There is lots of sex available even when a female is not in estrus, so there is little need for males to form coalitions to obtain sex. With every male out for himself, there is an opportunity for females to band together even though they are not related. Such alliances of females, along with their sociosexual behavior and bonding, enables them to monopolize food sources and keep themselves and their young safe from male attack. This alliance of females could only succeed if food sources were rich enough that individuals could feed together, rather than having to forage alone as chimpanzee females usually have to do in their environment. Bonobos live where there is extensive terrestrial herbaceous vegetation for the taking (Malenky and Wrangham, 1994), as well as huge abundant fruiting trees that can accommodate many feeding individuals. This behavioral and ecological situation that made females dominant also affected the males who were their sons. If a female were high-ranking, it made sense for her son to stay near her to share her high status. Groups of bonobos traveling through the forest became not male and female associates, but mother and son alliances.

CHIMPANZEES

There is sometimes a long-term bond between adult male chimpanzees and their mothers, although it is less strong than in bonobos. For example, on one occasion when her son Figan was 23 years old, Flo heard him cry in pain because he had hurt his wrist in a tussle with another male (Goodall, 1986). Although she was now old, she rushed 500 meters (550 yds) to be with him. He was still wailing when she arrived, so she sat down and groomed him. Thanks to her comfort, his screams soon diminished.

In the Mahale Mountain M group, the female Wanaguma, who had a cataract in one eye, hung out often with her only known son, the prime male NT. At the time, she was well into her forties and no longer breeding (Huffman, 1990). Sometimes the two of them traveled together apart from their group, and often she mixed with the other males with whom he was friendly. She seemed to associate with other chimpanzees, but this was largely because they kept close to her son NT, as did she. She groomed him and other chimpanzees occasionally, but he groomed her far more often.

In general for the M group, the few mothers with mature sons tended to stay near their sons when the mothers were not in estrus or were in semi-estrus, the son grooming his mother more than she groomed him. When the mother was in full estrus, however, and often soliciting copulations from other males, the son seldom interacted with her (Takahata, 1990a). Any attempt by a son to mate with his mother was very rare. For the M group, only one forced copulation was observed, that of 11-year-old TB of his mother (Nishida, 1990). She had been fishing for ants in a tree and after he attacked her she pushed him away so that he fell to the ground; he never tried to do that again. At Gombe, the exceptions were Satan and Goblin, even though their mothers usually objected to their advances, screaming and trying to escape.

In their report of chimpanzee (*Pan troglodytes verus*) behavior in the Taï forest of Ivory Coast in Africa, Christophe Boesch and his wife Hedwige Boesch-Achermann (2000) describe the adventures of Ella and her three sons Kendo, Fitz, and Gérald. They were usually together, so their family ties were strong; Fitz, for example, chose to remain with his mother until he was 13 years old. Kendo, the eldest, was anxious to defeat old Falstaff; when Kendo screamed at him, Ella rushed up followed by her younger sons, all barking, to support Kendo. Quickly Kendo became dominant to Falstaff. Ella and her two younger sons started to hang out with the male group to be near Kendo, who was then third in the male hierarchy order. Kendo began harassing the second-ranking male, Macho, with Ella's help. On three occasions in 1987, Ella herself attacked Macho, at which Kendo rushed to join her and together they chased Macho off. For the first time, Kendo was able, because his mother was present, to eat a red colobus monkey without Macho trying to take it away. When Ella was absent, however, Kendo left Macho alone. Eventually Macho (despite his name) became so conscious of Ella that he screamed whenever he heard her supportive bark, even if she was not in sight. At last in 1989, Kendo and Macho had a decisive battle that Kendo won. The alpha male, Brutus, had retired by this time with little resistance, so Kendo became, thanks to Ella's support, the dominant and most aggressive male that the researchers had seen. Ella died in 1990, while Fitz and Gérald, who had watched and learned from Kendo's battles, stayed on with the male group. The next year Kendo allowed Fitz himself to become alpha male to his beta status. Ella's behavior had rocketed her sons to a great height in a short time, indicating the importance of the mother–son relationship.

WOOLLY SPIDER MONKEYS OR MURIQUIS

In the Atlantic rainforest of south-east Brazil, researcher Karen Strier (1992) was teaching two assistants how to identify members of a troop of endangered woolly spider monkeys or muriquis (*Brachyteles arachnoides*) so they could help her in her behavioral research. (The excessively friendly nature of all those in the troop will be discussed in the chapter: *Family and group tight bonds*). The helpers needed to recognize each of about 30 animals individually to enable them to record all interactions among them. The three were sitting beside a trail in the morning, waiting for the monkeys in the trees above them to begin their day. Strier began to quiz the assistants on the identity of those visible in the foliage above. "Diego," they said correctly as they focused on one adult male. When a female swung over beside him, they studied her for a minute before correctly announcing that this was Didi. The students were not fazed by this, but Strier was. She had first seen Diego when he was an infant in 1982; now he was a healthy nine-year-old adult, and Didi was his mother. Mother and son exchanged a long, leisurely embrace. Then Didi settled down on a branch beside her son.

Strier was thrilled to see Didi and Diego together. When Diego had been an infant, so had Nilo, the son of Nancy. Diego and Nilo had both grown up in the troop, but whereas Diego now hung out with the adult males, Nilo spent much of his time with his mother and the adolescents. Strier wondered why Nilo behaved in this rather abnormal way. Was it because when he was five years old, he injured his arm in a fall and favored it for weeks afterward? Did this disrupt his normal social development, making him perhaps more reliant on his mother? Was he more cautious because of this and less able to be sociable with the other adult males? Or was it because Nancy had been more protective of her son than Didi had been? She had allowed her son to suckle until her next offspring was born, whereas Didi had not. Maybe the reason Nilo remained close buddies with his mother was simply a matter of the personality he had inherited.

COYOTES

Marc Bekoff, who has studied coyotes (*Canis latrans*) for more than 25 years, reports that it is not uncommon to see a female coyote hanging out with her adult son (personal communication, May 29, 2009). Where food is plentiful such as at Jackson Hole, Wyoming, coyotes live in family packs that can bring down a wounded or old elk (Lott, 2002), but there is great variation in their social organizations, and in most areas there are no long-term packs (Gier, 1975). Because of their smaller size, coyotes are unable to pull down large healthy prey animals as wolves do, so there is little need for a pack structure. Instead, they hunt as loners and in pairs (given their social nature), searching for such things as small mammals, birds, carrion, insects, and fruit.

LEOPARDS

Leopards (*Panthera pardus*) are thought to be solitary animals, but this is not always the case. During his research on the behavior of predators on the Serengeti plains of Africa, Brian Bertram (1978) put a radio collar on a healthy young male leopard of two and a half to three years of age. He was fully independent and well able to provide meat for himself. Nevertheless, he often joined forces at night with a lone old female whom Bertram suspected was his mother. The son seemed more keen on their friendship than did the mother; he would run after her, rub his flank along her side, give her a nudge with his rump, and rest his tail on her back. She seldom responded, although they did groom each other's head and neck sometimes. When the son's radio collar stopped working, Bertram lost track of this pair of leopards.

In his book *The Leopard*, Peter Turnbull-Kemp (1967) also mentions mothers and their grown sons hanging out together. He writes that when a mature male and a mature female are shot while feeding at a kill or bait, they are assumed to be a pair; instead, they are normally a mother and her grown son who has had only his mother as a lifelong companion. Rarely, such a duo may become man-eaters. In her book *Maasai Days*, Cheryl Bentsen (1989) also reports that a Maasai hunter told her that male and female leopards often travel in pairs that are likely mother and son.

PROVIDING FREE FOOD

Without the provisioning of chimpanzees and bonobos that was carried out by early scientists such as Jane Goodall, Toshisada Nishida, and Takayoshi Kano, we would know less about the behavior of these species than we do. What are the pros and cons of providing wild animals with nourishment they would otherwise not have? First, let us consider case studies of supplying free meals to chimpanzee, bonobo, and langur monkey groups.

When Goodall began her observations of chimpanzees in the forests of Gombe, Tanzania in 1961, she was frustrated at the difficulty of even seeing individual chimpanzees, let alone watching their interactions with others. She spent weeks and months following after them without much success. It seemed natural, then, to decide that if she could not get near the chimpanzees, she could perhaps lure them to her camp area by offering bananas at a feeding site, as she did in 1962. She and fellow workers soon came to recognize individuals and were able to collect amazing information, over a period of fifty years, on individual activities, behavior among group members, and interactions among the various groups that came to feed. Between 1964 and 1967, the bananas were attracting chimpanzees from several communities so that fights would often break out that would not otherwise have occurred (Goodall, 1986); at one point, 600 bananas were offered each day, enough to provide 40 percent of the caloric needs of an entire community (Ghiglieri, 1988). From 1968 on, only a few bananas every week were given to each chimpanzee who visited the food site, either alone or with a few companions, so that the aggression and the numbers who bothered to come fell markedly.

When Kano started his bonobo research in Zaire in 1973, like Goodall he provided food for the apes as he had done while researching the behavior of snow monkeys in Japan (de Waal, 1997); in order to entice the bonobos out of the forest and win their trust, he planted several hectares of sugar cane at the Wamba Forest site where he settled down. At Wamba, researchers were careful to offer food in only modest amounts and for only a few months of the year. When fruits from a number of trees were available, the bonobos preferred them anyway (Kano, 1992). During the research at Wamba, the number of bonobos and their health improved markedly, but Kano believes this was caused not by excess provisioning, but because the local people were interested in the research and so stopped injuring and threatening the animals. (There is no doubt that populations can sky-rocket

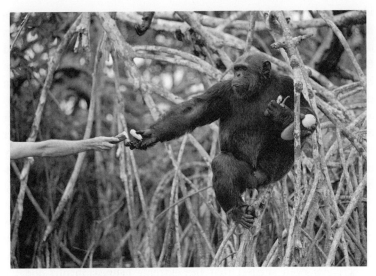

Figure 5. Unfortunately, feeding wild animals changes their behavior.
© photolibrary.com.

with too much artificial feeding, which is what happened in Japan to
Japanese macaques. As we have noted earlier, eventually there were so
many monkeys annoying farmers that to keep them from being shot, a
large number was sent to Texas to start a new colony of monkeys there
[Fedigan, 1991].)

Sarah Blaffer Hrdy (1977) in her book *The Langurs of Abu*, docu-
ments the behavior of langurs living in the town of Abu and its surroundings in north-west India. They hung out in fairly large troops of
two kinds: adult females with their young and one (rarely two) adult
male, and a looser group of young and mature males, with the exact
composition of troops constantly changing. Hrdy was able to recognize
many individuals, often by their nonconformities – hence the names
Harelip, Scrapetail, Splitear, Pawless, Righty Ear, Scarface, Slash-neck,
etc. that she gave to individuals. The langurs survived happily among
the Hindu people by swinging down from rooftops to snatch morsels
set out by priests, stealing food from the bazaar, or raiding garden
crops. Besides these various food sources, Hrdy also provided bananas
for them to eat on occasion. Competition for these tidbits caused a high
level of aggression and changes in hierarchy relationships among the
langurs, particularly during a season of drought when natural food was
limited.

The upside for scientists of offering free food is, of course, that
individual animals can be habituated to people more quickly and

identified by researchers so that data can be accumulated and published more rapidly. What about the down side? Provisioning members of the three species could have affected their friendly relationships. Did free food draw animals together as they fed? Or would individuals have been more friendly toward each other had they not fought over extra provisions? Would there be a looser dominance hierarchy or no hierarchy at all under natural non-provisioned conditions? If animals eat extra food set out for them that is not natural, it will not only affect their diet but also likely minimize the size of their ranges (because they may curtail their foraging in order to take advantage of the free handouts), increase the size of groups (as more individuals stay around because of the extra food available), affect hierarchy (if the dominant individuals are able to grab most of the food) or the sex ratio (if males manage to snatch more food than the smaller females), and increase aggression (which occurred because of fights over the food). Some researchers even suggest that the extreme aggression of Goodall's male chimpanzees may have been caused by provisioning (Wrangham, 1974), as may the battles for territory which killed a number of individuals (de Waal, 1997).

The problem with providing free food is that it is not possible to know what changes it has caused in a population, or how accurately a description of behavior for provisioned groups reflects the natural (non-provisioned) behavior of such animals. Hrdy argues on behalf of her research that for langur and rhesus monkeys, feeding by Hindu people (either directly or indirectly) has been done for at least several thousands of years, and thus has become a normal part of their existence.

Most extremely, David Hill (2004) argues that although rhesus monkeys and Japanese macaques have been studied under free-range conditions for 50 years, the collected data "are inadequate to allow a methodical assessment of the influence of demographic variation on kinship structure and behavior." This is because most of the information has come from animals that were provisioned. By feeding the monkeys, researchers have been able to collect data for scores of research articles, but Hill believes their conclusions may be misleading because they do not necessarily apply under non-provisioned natural conditions. Most acutely, provisioning has had a profound effect on the size and composition of macaque groups and on such processes as fission, all of which impact kin networks.

What about *not* provisioning a group of bonobos or chimpanzees? Researchers can be certain that the behavior of their subjects is more natural (although the very presence of people may affect the animals), but the work of habituating the apes to human observers can be onerous. Barbara Fruth and Gottfried Hohmann who studied the bonobos of Lomako, Zaire without offering them food, needed three years to be more or less accepted by the animals (de Waal, 1997). During that time, they could watch units feeding in large fruit trees, but when the animals came to the ground they quickly fled. It was impossible to collect many data on social friendships and interactions. They had much less obvious success there than did Kano (1992) at his provisioned Wamba location where research on bonobos had begun at about the same time.

Michael Ghiglieri (1988) had a better experience with his non-provisioned research program to study the behavior of chimpanzees in the Kibale forest of Uganda. Everyone had told him that he would fail, that it was impossible to study chimpanzees this way because they were able to move too quickly through the canopy and because they were frightened of poachers who sometimes hunted and killed them. (By contrast, orangutans and mangabeys can readily be followed because scientists can walk below them on the ground faster than they can travel in the trees.) Ghiglieri's successful *modus operandi* for his two-year research program was to observe over 100 large fruiting trees in the reserve, usually giant fig trees, find out when each was fruiting, and then sit each day about one hundred meters (110 yards) from the tree and watch with binoculars as groups of chimpanzees clambered through the branches stuffing themselves with the fruit. The figs often had wasps in them, which were a good source of protein. Ghiglieri sat still at first as if to hide, but was not upset if a chimpanzee spotted him; he then began to scratch himself as the chimpanzees often did, and they soon learned that although his behavior might seem odd, he meant them no harm. He was able to watch chimpanzees interact freely with each other with the exception of most females with infants; only two of these were unafraid of him enough to act naturally when he was nearby. In addition, he had no data on kinship among the animals because his work was too short-term. Ghiglieri was soon tolerated by many chimpanzees; his record day was seeing 34 of the 46 chimpanzees he knew by name feeding in the same huge fig tree, along with ten chimpanzees of whom he had little record. Non-provisioning worked fairly well for him.

In this chapter, we have seen that mothers and sons may live in the same group and thrive, allogrooming and hunting together, with the mother sometimes lending status to her offspring in fights for dominance. The question of researchers offering free food to attract their subjects remains controversial. To provision or not to provision? Each research team has to decide for itself which path to follow. Each has advantages and disadvantages, but not to provision is natural and best.

Fathers and their adult sons rarely live in the same group, but if they do, they have somehow to overcome their rivalry as mating partners for females. The following chapter discusses this issue and also that of grooming. Questions considered are why do dyads groom each other in some species but not in others? Why do some individuals groom their friend more than they are groomed in return? What does allogrooming or allopreening signify?

Fathers and sons, and social grooming and preening

In most social species, it is the adolescent males who leave their natal group to join another, which prevents inbreeding. A son who remains in his natal group with his father may cause tension because the two rivals both want to mate with the females in estrus. However, in at least two species, mountain gorillas and lions, some fathers and sons have been comrades. This chapter highlights information about social grooming, which is especially important in many of the higher primates. This activity is significant in cementing friendships between a dyad, indicating social relationships to other members of a community, and, of course, combatting parasites.

MOUNTAIN GORILLAS

Beethoven, the alpha male of group 5, was living with four adult females and various young when Dian Fossey (1983) first encountered the group in 1968. The dominant female was Effie and it was her first infant, Icarus, who developed a strong bond with his father while growing up in this polygamous family. The members of the group did everything together: travel through montane forests and open regions to areas of food, rest in a bunch at midday, play and groom as feelings allowed, seek protection together from pelting rain, and build sleeping nests for the night. At first, Icarus spent all of his time with his mother, but as the months and years passed he became a fully fledged member of the group in his own right. He began to help take on the male role of group protector against other gorillas and poachers. When Icarus was 11 years old, he was still immature but eager to mount young Pantsy when she was in estrus. Like many human fathers, Beethoven did not like this; when he saw them getting together he would run at them and whack them apart before mounting Pantsy himself.

In 1976, when Icarus was 14 and Beethoven about 47 years old, there was a violent battle between their group and a neighboring one. Fossey did not see the fight, but could follow its trail in the form of blood on the ground, torn out tufts of gorilla hair, pools of diarrhetic feces, and broken branches. At the end of the trail were her wounded friends: Beethoven had his arm so injured that the head of his humerus was visible, with torn ligaments and tendons around it; Icarus had eight deep bite marks on his head and arms. Beethoven was getting too old to defend his group on his own, so Icarus had obviously been an important supporter. For several weeks, the two males recuperated from the fight, resting together during the day, "exchanging soft belch vocalizations as though in mutual commiseration of their injuries." Icarus recovered much sooner than Beethoven, who took six months to heal completely. Icarus would leave his father to feed himself, then sometimes rush through the rest of the troop, threatening Pantsy especially, and her infant son, Banjo.[1] Icarus was now capable of mating with the females and, in theory, could have challenged his father for leadership of the group, but he did not do so.

The two silverbacks made an effective team in times of danger, Beethoven leading their group and Icarus bringing up the rear. Together, the two learned to scatter clusters of tourists and their armed guards who began to flood into the area to observe the gorillas made famous by Fossey's work. They made bluff charges that gave the invaders much to boast about when they returned home. Fossey, too, was enraged by these uninvited voyeurs and especially a French film crew that relentlessly badgered the animals for six weeks, day after day, to obtain footage for television. The trauma caused Effie to miscarry.

By the early 1980s Beethoven was no longer interested in females, so Icarus took over the function of mating with females of group 5. Icarus may seem like a model son, but to human eyes, he behaved bizarrely on several occasions. When Marchessa, one of the group females, died, he spent hours in frenzied attack upon her body. He pounded on it with his hands, leapt on it with both feet, and struggled to drag it about; Beethoven did little to stop his frenetic behavior. By contrast, the other group members tried to rouse the body by gentle means such as putting a finger or tongue in Marchessa's mouth or anus. Later Icarus, along with several of the females, fiercely attacked the orphaned infant Bonne Année whom Fossey was trying to introduce into their group. At one point, he grabbed the infant with his teeth and ran with her into the vegetation, only dropping her when Beethoven and several others charged after him. When Fossey finally managed to rescue the tiny animal and bring her up into the tree where she and a guide were crouched, Icarus and a female, Tuck, kept hostile guard below for over an hour before finally allowing them to escape. (Bonne Anneé successfully joined another group but died of pneumonia a year later.)

Not all father and son gorillas get along. Over the years, Fossey also watched another male–son combination in group 8, Rafiki and his son Samson, but they were so incompatible that Rafiki eventually drove Samson out of the family. When Rafiki died of old age, deeply mourned by Fossey, there was no silverback son to succeed him and so group 8 also perished.

LIONS

As we have seen, male lions are highly social with as many as four or more forming close bonded groups; the more of them there are, the more likely that they will be able to vanquish the male group already with a pride of females and become pride males themselves, eager to mate with the females. How do males hook up in order to form such a group? Extensive, long-term records dealing with the behavior and lineage of lion prides in the Ngorongoro Crater and the Serengeti, Tanzania, show that although it was uncommon, occasionally a son did join one or two males including his father (Packer and Pusey, 1982). Such an incorporation, which increased the size of the group, was known or suspected in four cases. Sons, therefore, in a few cases at least, join their father and perhaps other relatives to take on the adult role of males in lion society. However, incorporating younger relatives such as sons was never seen for male groups numbering three or more; one group of three male relatives actually prevented three younger relatives (sons and nephews) from joining them. Presumably, in large coalitions there are already enough males to prevent a take-over by another male group; even if the possible new-comer is a son who shares many of the genes of one or more pride males, his addition will still statistically decrease the number of matings for the others in the group.

SOCIAL GROOMING AND PREENING

Social grooming does not take place between individuals in all social species, or between all animals in a population, but when it does occur, it shows that these two friends who involve themselves in each other's care have an amiable relationship, and possibly a great one. Depending on the species, it may also be vital in delineating the social relationship of the two individuals for others in a community. Most furred or feathered animals autogroom (mammals) or autopreen (birds), which means tending to their own skin, fur, or feathers, while in a much smaller number of species, individuals groom each other as well (social grooming or allogrooming). In virtually all primate species, individuals show strong preferences for particular partners with whom to groom (Cheney and Seyfarth, 1990). This enables each to have a friend attend to areas of their body, such as around the head and neck, that are hard to see and reach. Social grooming is widely present in higher primates who have fingers with which to search adeptly through fur, but it can also be accomplished by teeth; in some lemurs, teeth have evolved into fine-toothed combs for raking through fur, indicating the importance of this activity. Allogrooming is present also in species of rodents, rabbits, and bats as well as in larger animals.

Allogrooming in primates

Allogrooming is especially important in primates because it functions, in part, as a social lubricant. In a literature survey of 44 species of free-living primates, Robin Dunbar (1991) found that only five, all of them arboreal, had not been seen to allogroom: the orangutan, a leaf monkey, a capuchin monkey, and two gibbon species. Allogrooming is a time-consuming activity so it must be important to animals, even as it is important to people who spend time and money at barbers, hairdressers, spas, and massage parlors.

Although grooming itself evolved originally for hygienic purposes (removal of dirt and dead skin) and to combat external parasites, which can seriously debilitate an individual by causing infections and loss of blood, it is practiced far more often in many species than would be necessary just to control lice, fleas, and ticks. In these species, it is important also in social ways when one individual grooms another. To relax while a friend gently manipulates one's skin is surely pleasurable; indeed, grooming between dyads of talapoin monkeys (*Miopithecus talapoin*) increases beta-endorphin concentrations in the cerebrospinal fluid, which in turn increases their feelings of social attachment (Keverne *et al.*, 1989). In addition, research has shown that a pigtail macaque groomed by another monkey had his heart rate fall by up to 20 beats per minute (Boccia *et al.*, 1989). Being groomed by a partner implies great trust on the part of both animals; either is in a vulnerable position should the other turn nasty.

Possible negative effects of grooming include a loss of water and electrolytes via saliva and tooth wear (Connor, 1995), and reduced resting time and vigilance for predators by both members of the dyad (Manson *et al.*, 2004). One research study showed that when the infants of rhesus monkeys wandered away, the mothers who were involved with grooming their partners paid less attention to them, with the result that these young were subject to increased abuse and harassment from other community members (Maestripieri, 1993). Rarely, if a groomee would rather not be groomed, this activity drives up tension rather than releasing it, with the groomee sometimes attacking his or her partner (Goosen, 1987).

For primate species that have a dominance hierarchy, allogrooming has been correlated with dominance ranking, especially for females who are generally more into grooming than males (Nakagawa, 1992):

- high-ranking adult females usually receive more grooming than do low-ranking ones,
- most grooming takes place between adult females of adjacent rank, if a dominance hierarchy exists,
- high-ranking adult females have more grooming partners than do low-ranking ones, and
- related adult females groom each other more than do non-related females.

The amount of time spent allogrooming varies greatly between individuals in a group, between groups themselves, and between species in the same genus; it is not obviously correlated with particular ecological or lifestyle characteristics (Goosen, 1987). Robin Dunbar (1991), who was puzzled about this question of why there was much more grooming in one species than another, researched several possibilities. Was the frequency of this activity carried out within a population related to the size of the monkeys' or apes' group? Was it a function of the area of surface skin of individuals (which, conveniently, is proportional to body weight, which can readily be estimated or taken)? Was it because, in larger groups, there is more chance of contagion of parasites and therefore more necessity for grooming?

Dunbar discovered that most social grooming occurred among the largest monkey populations, which were of Guinea baboons average group size (240 individuals), gelada baboons (113 individuals), and hamadryas baboons (51 individuals). The frequency of social grooming, therefore, was correlated with group size, especially in Old World monkeys. It was not correlated with individuals' body size. He thought that contagion of parasites was probably not important, because grooming time did not correlate well with group size in New World monkeys the way it did with Old World species. Dunbar suggested that because only Old World species make extensive use of complex social strategies, such as deception and formation of group alliances, perhaps social grooming was related to their more complex brains.

Dunbar then teamed up with H. Kudo (Kudo and Dunbar, 2001) to study the connection between grooming, sociality, and increased brain size. They found that the size of the neocortex of the brain correlated positively with the size of grooming cliques in 30 species of non-human primates. Presumably, there is an upper limit on the size of groups within which primates can socialize adequately; when a group becomes larger than this, it will become less stable, less coherent, less functional, and may eventually break into several smaller groups.

Robert Barton (1985), in his research, focused on where on his or her body a primate groomed and was groomed by a friend, observing 19 different species of primates living in zoos to make this project feasible. The species included chimpanzees, gibbons, Old World and New World monkeys, and lemurs. He classified 17 areas of the body as being either "accessible" or "inaccessible." The latter were the face, head, neck, upper back, middle back, lower back or tail base, and anogenital region or ischial callosities; most of these areas could be reached by hand, but an animal could not scan them visually. Lemurs who groom with their teeth are physically unable to reach their own head and neck areas. Barton hypothesized that if allogrooming had an important utilitarian function, it should be concentrated on body areas of a groomee that were inaccessible to that individual.

From his observations, Barton found that this was so; although inaccessible places were in smaller areas on the animals than accessible ones, all the species studied had an overwhelming concentration of allogrooming on these sites. Grooming does, therefore, have a utilitarian purpose facilitated to some extent by the groomee, who often presents to the groomer hard-to-reach areas in particular need of attention. Groomers are willing to oblige their friend for various reasons:

(a)   grooming serves as a positive social interaction between the dyad, so it should be harmonious and sensitive for the groomee,

(b)   hygienically efficient grooming is probably favored by kin selection where the partner is closely related,

(c)   inefficient grooming might be devalued for possible later reciprocation by the groomee, and

(d)   the groomer will benefit by grooming an area with many parasites if he or she considers them as a food supplement. Animals in the wild who do not have a friend with whom to groom reciprocally have been seen to be infested with parasites, especially in inaccessible parts of their body.

How to tell a partner where you itch? In talapoin monkeys, a female approaches another while exposing her groin or chest area with legs or arms spread apart and head turned aside. By lowering her head, she indicates that one of these is the preferred area. If she wants her back groomed, she crouches down or lies prostrate near her friend (Keverne *et al.*, 1989).

The importance of social grooming, which can occupy up to 20 percent of the daily time budget, has attracted great interest recently as possible "currency." If one monkey grooms another, will he or she be groomed for a similar length of time ("time-matching"), thus equalizing services? Could the service be remembered and time-matched later on? Could grooming be reciprocated by some other service, such as an alliance for combat? Peter Henzi and Louise Barrett (1999) argue against the possibility that allogrooming is mainly to obtain support for competitive interactions among monkeys – the "grooming for aid" hypothesis. They propose instead, for female primates – and show that this is true in two populations of chacma baboons (*Papio ursinus*) in South Africa – that individuals either trade their grooming for being groomed in return or for greater tolerance toward them by more dominant animals. This tolerance could take the form of reduced aggression, increased access to scarce resources, or increased tolerance around infants whom many adults love to touch or handle. In species such as chimpanzees, where females rather than males emigrate from their natal troop at puberty, it is the males who have known each other since their youth who have extensive interchanges between grooming given and other support received (Watts, 2002).

Joseph Manson and his colleagues (2004) delved into this topic further, providing new information on the subject for white-faced capuchins (*Cebus capucinus*) and bonnet macaques (*Macaca radiata*). They conclude from data for dyads of these species, along with data from baboon dyads, that a variety of forces can influence grooming dynamics. Some grooming triggers reciprocal grooming, the grooming itself being parceled into small episodes so that a monkey will not be "cheated" by providing extensive grooming that is not then reciprocated. A male may groom a female more when she is in estrus; or an animal's status may itself be heightened when he or she is seen grooming an individual higher in the hierarchy. Far more information about grooming must be collected and analyzed from many more species before all of these factors can be analyzed and fully understood.

To illustrate the role of both social grooming and autogrooming in removing parasite eggs, Koichiro Zamma (2002) tallied the number of louse eggs on eight carcasses of wild Japanese monkey females shot as agricultural pests. When the bodies were removed from the freezer, he measured squares one cm by one cm (0.155 sq in) on nine different areas of each body in which he counted the number of hairs. In a larger square 4 cm by 4 cm (0.62 sq in), he counted all the eggs belonging to two species of lice (*Pedicinus obtusus* and *P. eurygaster*) on the same nine body areas – there were almost no other ectoparasites present.

Zamma also video-taped the grooming behavior of wild Japanese monkeys of the E group at Arashiyama, Kyoto, both while focal animals were grooming themselves and grooming a friend. From the tapes, he counted the duration of these sessions, the number of hand–stroke movements, and the number of movements needed to remove a louse egg from each of the nine body areas. This last action involved the groomer pulling up the egg along a hair with the nail of her first finger and the tip of her thumb, then touching her finger and/or thumb to her lips. (The eggs are presumably tastier than we might think.) Zamma estimated from his measurements that there were, on average, about 550 louse eggs on a monkey and about 3.9 million hairs, but these were not randomly distributed. Most of the louse eggs as well as most of the hairs were on the outer sides of the body with few on the chest, inner arms, and belly.

The videotapes showed that the monkeys groomed both themselves and others a total of 74,782 strokes during the research, with 1594 movements to remove louse eggs. Most of this activity was aimed at the outer areas of the bodies where there were the most hairs and the most parasitic eggs. Because the outer areas with more hairs were groomed for longer, with more eggs removed by the groomer, grooming was not random but rather geared toward sites with dense hair.

These monkeys seem doomed to be lice-ridden forever, as lice continue to lay about six dozen eggs a day on a monkey who, along with a friend, continues to try to eradicate them. The number of eggs will probably not decrease, but will not skyrocket either. Zamma estimates that if a monkey stopped grooming and being groomed, the number of louse eggs in her (or his) fur would increase by a factor of two in one week, and by a factor of 30 in a month. Because she needs to be groomed daily to prevent such infestation, particularly in body areas that she cannot reach very well herself, such as her upper back, she must form a social bond with a friend to do this. Indeed, it is best that she have several grooming partners in case one dies or is injured. Zamma concludes that one of the important reasons Japanese monkeys live in groups is to keep their bodies clean: "the hygienic function of allogrooming, which is naturally an altruistic behavior, simultaneously fulfills a social function."

Allogrooming in non-primates

We have noted previously that social grooming occurs in horses, and it is present in other non-primate species, too. Impala (*Aepyceros melampus*) living in tick-infested woodland areas of Africa are especially plagued with these parasites. From a vehicle, Benjamin Hart and Lynette Hart (1992) watched large herds of these antelope in Kenya, noting down grooming sessions that occurred when one impala approached or turned toward another. Allogrooming began when one animal made upward sweeping movements, called episodes, of the "lateral dental grooming apparatus" (comprising the lower incisors and canine teeth whose functional shape evolved presumably for this purpose) or the tongue against the lie of the fur on the neck or head of his or her partner. Each episode lasted about a second. On average, about six to 12 grooming episodes made up a bout, and these were exchanged between the two animals, tit for tat, until one partner perhaps changed to another area of the body. An encounter was defined as the exchange of bouts until one partner stopped grooming. Richard Connor (1995) refers to this as the "parcelling model of reciprocity" which keeps "cheating" to a minimum.

Most encounters in impala groups were between two females, with the longest of all being 44 exchanges with 21 bouts and 23 bouts. Rarely, about five percent of the time, one animal gave two "gratuitous" bouts sequentially before receiving a bout. Most episodes involved teeth rather than tongue even when the grooming occurred in the eye region. The Harts found no suggestion of solicitation by any animal; the grooming just started when one animal began it. During the allogrooming, the groomee might lower, raise, or turn her head to expose to the groomer skin areas that needed attention. Although a territorial male kept company with the females and their young, on only five occasions did an

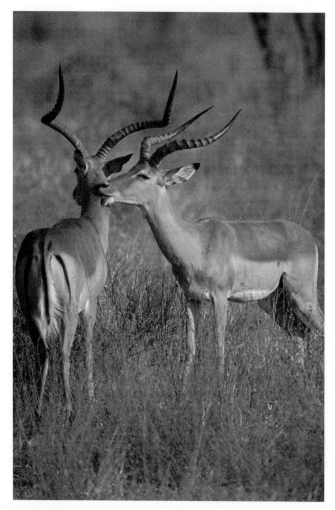

Figure 6. Bachelor male impala groom each other.
© photolibrary.com

adult female and this male allogroom, even though the males took little time to self-groom. On each occasion, the initial bout was given by the male, but on two of these, the female did not return the favor.

Allogrooming similar to that among the females also occurred between adult males in the bachelor groups; these encounters usually ended with the animals pressing their horns together or sparring lightly. Their allogrooming was also highly reciprocal. The Harts observed that either the smaller or larger (subordinate or dominant) of two impala could start the grooming, and did not know if any of the individuals involved were related.

In a second research project, the Harts and two other colleagues (1992) compared grooming behavior in the impala to that in three other Kenyan ungulates: Thomson's gazelle, Grant's gazelle, and wildebeest. These three species groomed themselves on the head and neck with a hoof, an activity reduced in impala who presumably allogroomed instead to rid themselves of ticks. In all four species, the territorial males groomed only about half as much as did the females and bachelor males, which reflects their need to be constantly vigilant in herding females and/or preventing rival males from taking over their territory. The impala reciprocal allogrooming strategy seems to be unique among wild antelope and other ungulates.

A few years later, Michael Mooring and his colleagues including Benjamin Hart (1996) addressed the question of tick load on impala during their breeding season in Zimbabwe. When some impala were shot to reduce their population, the researchers counted the numbers of larvae, nymphs, and adult ticks on the three different types of adults (female, bachelor male, and territorial male). They wanted to test two hypotheses: Do individuals that groom most harbor fewest ticks, which is the programmed-grooming hypothesis? Or do individuals who groom most harbor the most ticks, according to the stimulus-driven hypothesis? They found that territorial males (who groomed the least) had the most ticks, the females (who groomed the most) had the fewest, and the bachelor males (who had intermediate grooming) had an intermediate number of ticks. The results therefore supported the programmed-grooming hypothesis. The low grooming rate of males compared to females was attributed to their greater vigilance and rutting behavior, and/or to high testosterone levels that act to suppress oral grooming. Either way, by seldom grooming and never allogrooming, a territorial male may suffer a significant cost to his well-being and his reproductive activity – his territory and his mating possibilities usually lasted for less than four months before he was displaced by another male.

Allogrooming has been studied in a much smaller species too, the highly social Cape ground squirrel (*Xerus inauris*) of southern Africa. Melissa Hillegass and her colleagues (2008) researched this animal's parasite infestation in the wild because they wanted to know if the parasite load was correlated with group size, or with the species' social structure. They live-trapped the wild squirrels from 18 adult male and matrilineal female groups (comprising from one to nine females and their young). With a metal flea comb, each captured animal had his or her back and sides combed from the shoulders to the base of the tail so that all ectoparasites present (fleas, ticks, and lice) fell directly into an ethanol solution in a petri dish, which immediately killed them. Feces of each animal were also collected so that internal parasites could be counted. The squirrels were checked for body weight, sex, and reproductive condition before a small transponder was placed under their skin for permanent identification. Before release, each squirrel was also dye-marked and freeze-marked so he or she could be recognized from a distance. Because these ground squirrels are diurnal, living in open habitats with low vegetation, it is fairly easy to observe their activity from hides on the roof of vehicles or from observation towers. For four months the researchers recorded which individuals groomed and were allogroomed by which other individuals and for how long. They also mapped out the large home ranges of adult males and the smaller ones of females.

From their results, the scientists found that group size was not correlated with the number of parasites on their members, but that males carried about three times as many ectoparasites as females, while females harbored nearly three times as many endoparasites. All the animals self-groomed for about the same amount of time, but females allogroomed more than did males. They hypothesize that testosterone in the males may reduce resistance to ectoparasites as has been noted in other species, and that for females, their smaller home ranges and denser populations may increase their exposure to endoparasites. Allogrooming would presumably reduce ectoparasite loads, especially in females who allogroomed more, which would mitigate the cost of grouping. They do not speculate about whether allogrooming has a role in bonding or socializing individuals, which would be difficult to prove.

It is impossible to carry out field observations of grooming in very small animals such as mice and shrews, so here we shall consider only one captive species. Pavel Stopka and Romana Graciasova (2001) studied the non-aggressive herb-field mouse (*Apodemus microps*) in the Czech Republic using surveillance videocameras to document grooming and allogrooming in wild-caught mice under experimental conditions. They found that self-grooming was stereotypic, lasted about eight seconds, and was done at random even in the absence of parasites such as ticks and fleas. Allogrooming between two males or two females was reciprocal – maybe not immediately but in the long term. However, males groomed females longer than vice versa. This asymmetry probably reflects a similar trend in other rodents, where males are "generous" because they want to obtain information about a female's reproductive status and/or to establish a mating relationship. Social grooming is also present in some bats, such as the vampire bat, but it has only been studied in captive animals (Wilkinson, 1986).

Allopreening

Photographers trying to shoot brilliant bird portraits know the huge amount of time that their subjects spend preening their feathers in unphotogenic postures, oiling and realigning them incessantly. Preening involves nibbling at the base of feathers and running them through the bill. Few birds preen the feathers of another bird. As early as 1965, C. J. O. Harrison published a comprehensive survey of allopreening that is still authoritative today. He reported that 41 different taxonomic families of birds had at least one species in which allopreening had been observed, but that the vast majority of birds (given that there are 157 avian families and that allopreening may have been observed in only one or two species in a family) do not allopreen.

Allogrooming is used to cement social bonds between two individuals, but this is a minor use for allopreening, which is thought generally to be connected with aggression, the antithesis of friendship. Birds in general do not like to cosy up to one another, as is evident when one sees a line of starlings or pigeons perched along a telephone wire, spread out at equal intervals so that each bird's "individual space" is honored. If this space is invaded, as it is in colonial nesting birds and in breeding pairs when both adults are present at the nest, it often triggers hostility and allopreening, which is commonly done by the dominant or more aggressive bird, usually a male. Sometimes allopreening is so vigorous that the recipient jumps back as if hurt; in razorbills (*Alca torda*) who live in cliff colonies of thousands of nests, affectionate nibbling between a pair may degenerate into a savage fight that knocks one bird off the ledge; when she or he returns, the gentle allopreening may resume. Allopreening almost always occurs around the head or neck, where a bird under threat would be attacked by the beak of another. This attack possibility provokes a preening-invitation posture in the less aggressive bird, which involves squatting slightly while fluffing and raising the feathers on its neck and head, making it resemble a fledgling. This posture, in turn, triggers a gentle pecking reaction rather than an assault from the would-be aggressor.

How do we know that allopreening around the head and neck does not correspond with allogrooming in mammals, which serves to remove parasites from this same body area that the recipient cannot reach for itself? After all, it occurs especially in colonial nesting species where ectoparasites can easily spread from one bird to another. Harrison believed that it was not an anti-parasite device because:

(a)   allopreening rarely occurs on the torso where ectoparasites are also present;

(b)   allopreening is unknown in most species that also have parasites;

(c)   even in species in which allopreening is present, it may take place only in the breeding season whereas parasites thrive all year long; and

(d)   in some species, allopreening is too brief and limited to be of any use against parasites.

Harrison suggested that in species whose members form a pair-bond for life and are constantly in each other's company, allopreening might help to maintain pair-bonds between dyads, just as allogrooming does in mammals. This is true, for example, for crows and other species that have been studied recently. Andrew Radford and Morné du Plessis (2006) report that the cooperatively breeding green wood-hoopoe of South Africa (*Phoeniculus purpureus*) may be such a species, as well as one in which allopreening *does* reduce parasite loads. Over a period of many months, they watched six color-ringed groups (each of two to seven individuals) of these birds through binoculars to note all inter-actions between adults. They sexed birds by noting bill lengths and vocalizations, and determined dominance by displacement activity. Allopreening involved preeners making soft jabs of the bill at their partners or running their feathers through their bill. Birds were often caught so that the number of mites, fleas, and lice on their bodies could be counted – 0 indicated no parasites visible while 3 represented a heavy ectoparasite infestation.

The researchers found that infestation was high in wood-hoopoe groups because they roosted together in a tree cavity each night. All the birds allopreened each other in the head area, which reduced high parasite loads as well as serving a social function. It mostly benefited the breeding pair, dominant individuals who received more body (as opposed to head) allopreening than did other birds. If a dominant bird initiated an allopreening session, it was more likely to be reciprocated than if a subordinate bird did the initiating. Dominant birds also terminated more preening bouts than did subordinates.

Parrots that mate for life may also allopreen in order to maintain a strong pair-bond, as has been shown for the orange-fronted parakeet (*Aratinga canicularis*) year round and for Amazon parrots (*Amazona albifrons*) (Skeate, 1984). For Amazon pairs, allopreening is confined to the head and neck region. The soliciting bird lowers its head toward its consort with its feathers ruffled. Once its partner begins to preen in response, the solicitor changes the angle or position of its head to indicate which new areas should be addressed. Solicitation of preening also seems to be used to appease or soothe an agitated mate.

Sue Lewis and her associates (2007) carried out a study on allopreening in common guillemot (*Uria aalge*) on an island in the Firth of Forth, Scotland. There each paired female lays a single egg on a cliff ledge, which she and her partner incubate and where later they bring food to the nestling. Guillemot society is a model of togetherness, both temporal and physical. Individuals are long-lived, and nesting pairs so close together on a cliff face that birds may shift over to preen not only their partner, but also their neighbor. Because of this crowding, they are infested with seabird ticks (*Ixodes*). As research on this colony had been on-going for many years, it was already documented that the duration of the average pair-bond was nearly five years, while relationships between a bird and his or her neighbor lasted, on average, about one and a half years. To carry out their research, the scientists videotaped 33 pairs of guillemots, one or both members of whom were color-ringed so they could be told apart. The sex of each bird was established, in part by watching its behavior. From recording tapes they quantified the rates of allopreening during the incubation period and the number of social preenings and fights between neighbors.

Between pairs of guillemots, the male preened the female more than she did him, perhaps to stimulate the production of care-promoting hormones, such as prolactin. Both the males and females equally preened neighbors of either sex reciprocally, although pairs did so at different rates. The pairs who had the highest rates of allopreening with neighbors had a higher breeding success than other pairs. The combative lesser-allopreening pairs had more fights with their neighbors and less breeding success, which was especially apparent when an egg or chick was bumped or pushed off a ledge during a scuffle. Allopreening between partners may help maintain the social bond between the mated pair (how can this be measured?), while reciprocal allopreening between neighbors is important in reducing stress and fighting. Allopreening, which is concentrated in the head and neck areas, did indeed also reduce tick infestations, despite Harrison's report.

In summary, males and their adult sons almost never live in the same groups, but they have done so exceptionally in gorillas and lions. Grooming and sometimes allopreening in mammals and birds are important in cementing friendships between two compatible individuals.

This and earlier chapters have focused on different types of dyads. But friendship can be far more inclusive than this, encompassing all the members of a group so close-knit that it is impossible to pinpoint one or two duos as more ardent than others, as we shall see in the following chapter.

Family and group tight bonds

Some species are so social that it is impossible to say that any two or three individuals are closer psychically than any others. The family group is together all the time – togetherness that would drive most people mad. The three species represented here are the elephant, orca, and naked mole-rat. Other species have groups whose closeness depends upon their environment – if the area is densely populated with animals of the same species, then mature youngsters will not be able to start reproducing for themselves, but may stay with their natal family, helping to raise the next year's young. Examples are wolves, coyotes, beaver, crows, and gibbons. The final five species discussed, woolly spider monkeys, black-handed spider monkeys, lesser kudu, white rhinoceros, and sperm whales, form friendly groups for reasons that require further study.

ELEPHANTS

Are there preferred dyads, triads, foursomes, or any other combination of individuals present in maternal elephant troops? There is no way to tell. A herd of adult female elephants (*Loxodonta africana*) and their young (the males go their separate ways when they reach adolescence) is so tight that infants, nieces, mothers, aunts, grandmothers, and great-grandmothers are never really separated during their entire, long lives. Cynthia Moss, in her book *Elephant Memories* (1988), which she wrote after researching the social behavior of elephants in Amboseli National Park for 20 years, notes that all females and young live in such family units. Individuals coordinate their activities so that they are doing the same thing at the same time. If they are traveling, wallowing, resting, or standing, they tend to bunch closely together; they are immensely tactile, often touching each other with their trunks, or leaning and rubbing against one another. (What a nightmare this scenario would be for humans who value their independence!) If, during migration, a baby cannot keep up with the others, the adults slow down as they move forward; if an old female is sick or dying, they gather around her as if offering silent sympathy. When members of a herd have been feeding for a few hours somewhat apart, they salute each other fervently when they again join forces, raising their heads, spreading and flapping their ears, tucking in their chins, and rumbling loud and throatily. If herd members have been separated for a few days, their greetings are even more vehement. They may "spin around urinating and defecating and, with their heads and ears high, fill the air with a deafening cacophony of rumbles, trumpets, roars, and screams" (Poole, 1996). The intensity of the ceremony reflects the degree of their attachment.

The adult bulls usually form loose groups in which individuals, when they are in musth and sexually active, leave by themselves to find females in estrus with whom to copulate. When their period of musth is over, they return to the same group. Within these male groups (which may be composed of relatives) some individuals tend to hang out with a preferred friend much more often than others – some dyads are seen together rarely, but others as much as 36 percent of the time (Moss and Poole, 1983). A lone bull too old to keep up with his group sometimes retires along with a younger companion to a riverine area where soft vegetation is available that the oldster can eat with his worn teeth (see the chapter: *Old buddies*).

In his book *Elephant Life* (oddly named because the author was involved in elephant death, namely the slaughter of 200 Ugandan individuals), Irven Buss (1990) reports, ghoulishly, on close bonds between adult and young elephants, the tightest being between a matriarch and the first two filial generations. He notes that a matriarch exhibited "exceptionally aggressive behavior" when he "collected" (shot to death) her subadult son, and "equally aggressive behavior" when he "collected" her grandchild 17 days later.[1]

Retired female elephants from zoos and circuses do pair up when they are sent to an elephant sanctuary in Tennessee (CBS News, 2009/ 01/02). Co-founder Carol Buckley says that the animals arrive one by one, but tend to live out their lives two by two – for example, Debbie with Ronnie, and Misty with Dulary. "Every elephant that comes here searches out someone that she then spends most all of her time with. It's like having a best girlfriend. Someone they can relate to, they have something in common with." For an elephant, it is infinitely better than being friendless and alone.

ORCAS (KILLER WHALES)

Whales are different than many terrestrial social groups; they are not territorial (their foraging areas are so vast that no resource can be controlled), they are not monogamous, and the males do not provide paternal care to the young (Whitehead, 2003). Fellowship among social whales and dolphins is especially important for feeding:

(a)   individuals can join forces to chase and capture fish prey,

(b)   the behavior of individuals gives information to others about the presence of food,

(c)   if the fish prey escapes from one individual, another is likely to grab it, and

(d)   individuals can avoid feeding in an area being utilized by others.

Like elephant families, resident orcas (*Orcinus orca*) also live in closely bonded groups, but elephant males, like the males of most dolphin and whale species, leave their natal group when they reach maturity. By contrast, resident orca males (as well as pilot whale males) do not do so (Hoyt, 1990).[2] There seems to be no terrestrial counterpart to a species where all the young remain in their natal group throughout their lifespan and the males, to prevent inbreeding, mate with females from other groups when they encounter them (Connor and Peterson, 1994). A family of resident orcas is so closely bonded that members even breathe together, the blows of individuals occurring almost simultaneously. Peter Knudtson (1996) notes that "the rhythm of breathing could serve as a dramatic behavioural display of family unity, of social familiarity and even of affection among whales." A matrilineal group, the basis of resident orca society, is composed usually of three generations – the matriarch, her daughters and sons, and her daughters' offspring. If the group becomes too large, a daughter and her young may break away to form a new group. A number of family groups make up a pod, but there is no record of an individual ever changing groups within the pod. All members of a pod have the same dialect of vocalizations (listened to diligently by whale researchers using hydrophones), but subtle variations exist within each family.

There may be dyads of individuals who prefer to hang out with each other within a group, but how can we know this when it is so difficult to see them in the water? Perhaps there was a special bond between Top Notch and Foster, two big brothers living in the coastal waters of British Columbia, but perhaps I just hope this was so because of their sad story (Morton, 2002). One day they were seen swimming around Hanson Island, calling and calling. No one knew where the rest of their group was but when Eva, their mother, was found dead several days later, cast up on a nearby beach among drift wood, they realized that her sons had been calling for her. For the first time in their existence (Top Notch was then thirty-three), she was no longer there to answer them or share their lives.

NAKED MOLE-RATS

We know little about naked mole-rats (*Heterocephalus glaber*) because they inhabit underground burrows in dry regions of East Africa. Because of their environment, they are close-knit physically, up to 300 of them crawling over and under each other in their tunnels, carrying out a variety of tasks (Griffin, 2008). Individuals average about 10 cm in length (4 in), with only a few sensory hairs on their bodies, poor eyesight because they live in the dark, and short, thin legs that can propel them as fast backward as forward. They use their large protruding top incisors to dig through soil, their lips sealed behind the teeth so that dirt does not get into their mouths. The tubers and bulbs they discover during their digging become their chief source of food, along with their own feces.

To study their behavior, zoologists dug up almost a complete colony of the animals from a location in Kenya and transplanted them to an artificial burrow system in a laboratory setting where, after each of the 16 females and 24 males had been individually marked, they were left alone for a year to become organized in their new quarters. Then their activities were observed in detail. Jennifer Jarvis (1981) does not report if any two individuals were particularly friendly – this would be difficult to observe and prove little, given their artificial conditions.

Mole-rats are the only eusocial mammals known, eusociality being defined as having a social system with physically and/or physiologically distinct castes. Jarvis identified the castes as the sole, large breeding female and adult males (some breeding). Non-breeding females fitted into the categories of: (a) frequent workers, the smallest; (b) larger infrequent workers; and (c) nonworkers, the largest. The work of the breeding female is to produce young for the group (up to 28 pups in one litter!), and that of the workers to dig tunnels and a toilet area, transport food material to the communal nest, defend the colony, and care for the young. This arrangement is reminiscent of ant societies. The physical

closeness of mole-rats is emphasized by high levels of inbreeding determined from their DNA (Reeve *et al.*, 1990), and by their huddling behavior with the young to keep warm in winter because of their lack of hair.
Their lifestyle may seem restrictive, but it has its advantages (if that sort
of life appeals) in that individuals can live for 30 years, 15 times as long
as other mammals of about the same size (Griffin, 2008).

Parents and their helping offspring

Ideally, when the progeny of a breeding pair of animals grow to maturity, they go off to start their own families. Instead, in some cases, they
remain with their parents where they are relatively well protected,
working with them to raise their second brood, often a year later.
Stephen Emlen (1982), in his article "Ecological constraints of helping,"
describes two reasons why this is so. First, they may live in a stable
habitat already saturated with members of their species, so there is no
room or opportunity to set up a new family. Second, the environment
may be harsh and swiftly changeable (sudden droughts, floods), creat-
ing the functional equivalents of unpredictable breeding openings and
closures. When the chance for the young of reproducing successfully is
small enough, evolutionary selection will favor individuals who
remain as non-breeders within their natal groups; at least their efforts
to help raise their siblings will benefit their common DNA. Grown
offspring remain at home when the cost of leaving is prohibitive.

WOLF PACKS

Dogs and wolves (*Canis lupus*) are close enough genetically to be able to
interbreed, but their social behaviors are completely different. Male
dogs, during their long history of domestication, have learned to get
their sex where they can find it, with never a thought of being companions to the female or helping to raise her pups. By contrast, the
alpha wolf pair form a wonderful friendship that can last for years or a
lifetime, copulating each spring and supplying the yearly litter of pups
with all the necessities for growth and health. They are helped by the
rest of the pack, usually comprising their older offspring and other
relatives. The familial duties include caring for the young cubs, hunting for prey, and patrolling their territory. Bonding between the alpha
pair is strengthened physically and emotionally at matings, when they
are connected for half an hour or so by the copulatory tie (Busch, 2007).
The entire pack bonds together as they howl, thereby coordinating and

synchronizing activities such as travel movements and hunting. The wolves often urinate in sequence at the same spot, causing wolf researcher David Mech to remark that "Wolves that pee together stay together" (Zimen, 1981). (Companion dogs living together will do this too [Thomas, 1994].) Jeffrey Masson (1999) describes an alpha male in Alaska coming back from a pack hunt to the alpha female and their six small cubs. "The father walks straight up to the den, where he is greeted by his mate with enthusiastic wagging of her tail and moans and groans of pleasure: She is happy to see him return."

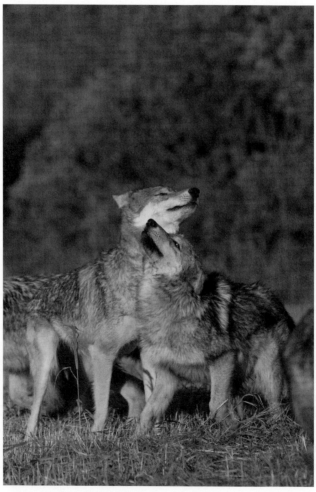

Figure 7. Wolves in packs are closely banded.
© istockphoto.com/Frank Parker

Douglas Smith and Gary Ferguson (2005) give a history of the Leopold Pack, the first Yellowstone pack in recent times named for Aldo Leopold, the noted environmentalist who first recommended in 1944 that wolves be reintroduced into this National Park from where they had been exterminated by human activity long before. The Leopold alphas were numbers 7 and 2, two of the 31 Canadian wolves transplanted there in 1995 to make Leopold's dream come true. After being acclimatized in a pen in the Park to ensure they would not head back home to Canada, number 7 was released, wearing a radio collar so that scientists could follow her wanderings. She spent her first ten months living successfully on her own before teaming up with number 2, to the excitement of the scientists following her progress. She was out killing elk only days before giving birth to three pups, which the wolf pair successfully raised, making the family a true pack.

Over the next seven years, Leopold Pack produced litters each spring, totaling 34 pups in all, at least 29 of whom survived beyond age one year – an amazing feat. Two of these offspring went on to form packs of their own. Numbers 7 and 2 had chosen an almost perfect territory for the pack; its boundaries have remained almost the same from 1996 to the present, and it was one of the few packs whose members never left the safety of the Park. For over six years during the tenure of numbers 7 and 2, Leopold Pack's size remained stable between 11 and 13 members, presumably the optimal number for the prey in the area; only the alpha pair bred each year, the yearly pups solicitously raised by all the pack wolves who were closely related genetically. When the pups were first born, pack members took turns baby-sitting them so they were never alone, and bringing food back to the den to feed them.

In May 2002, number 7 was killed by members of a neighboring pack; she was an old wolf by then, but still nursing the pups she had borne a month earlier. Leopold Pack rallied around to save these youngsters, feeding them bits of partially digested meat because they had no milk to give them. All eight survived. Number 2 died seven months later, no longer alpha male because of his great age, but Leopold Pack continues as an entity to this day.

Beyond the permanent bond between the alpha couple, Eric Zimen (1981) describes a sequence of temporary bonds based on genetics that govern much of wolf behavior, and roughly defined as existing between place or animals who tend to stay close together for much of the time. Initially, the pups are bonded to the den where they are born in the spring, and their mother is bonded to them. At this time, the den forms the core of the pack. When the pups are about three weeks old, this latter bond is so weakened that their mother begins to sleep outside rather than inside with them. By late August, the pups are quite big, independent, and a nuisance to their elders. By late fall, the pups are choosing to sleep near the adults rather than vice versa. They are then considered active members of the pack who may decide, during the winter, to leave or to remain in it.

John Theberge (1998) gives information in his book *Wolf Country* about wolf packs (*Canis lupus lycaon*)[3] in Algonquin Park, Ontario, where he and Mary Theberge, his wife whom I was fortunate to have had as a student, put radio collars on scores of individuals in order to keep track of their movements, territories, activities, and pack-memberships. Other methods yielding data included the Theberges howling at night to see who howled back (from which they could sometimes tell the pack the animals belonged to and their number); recording and mapping all tracks of deer, moose, beaver, and wolf they came across; collecting carcasses or parts of them from which to determine age and cause of death; and evidence of plant species browsed by deer and moose and to what extent, to determine the health of the prey population. Both Theberges worked relentlessly over 12 years to collect and analyze their data, canoeing for hours to reach inaccessible sites, swatting a myriad of black flies and mosquitoes, staying up all night to record wolf activity, and camping out in subzero weather.

The Theberges found that the closest alliance for a mated pair was between Jocko 3 (the female) and Basin 6 Jocko, who were never more than 100 meters apart during the many times their positions were monitored from an overhead plane or by nearby researchers over the course of a year and a half. Other pack members were close buddies too, although often spread out from the rendezvous site in search of prey or a carcass to scavenge. As well as the alpha pair, two males or two females sometimes foraged together, perhaps representing preferred friendships within the pack; with success, they would eat their fill and then fetch other members of the pack to eat as well.

Wolves are so gregarious that to come across a lone middle-aged wolf without a pack indicated to the researchers that something was very wrong. In the Algonquin Park case, the wrong was men shooting, as vermin, many of the Algonquin wolves when they left the park in autumn, following deer migrating south. After the slaughter of one alpha female, members of her pack repeatedly gave what the Theberges called the mourning howl – "long, forlorn notes breaking downward in melancholy intervals." This howl was given both by wolves in captivity and in the wild when a packmate was injured or killed. The death of an alpha animal was particularly devastating to a pack, which then often became dysfunctional to some extent, lacking as it did the experience and wisdom of this leader.

COYOTE PACKS

Coyotes (*Canis latrans*), who are so closely related to wolves that they may interbreed, also form packs where there is ample food in the form of large ungulates. Such packs can last for four years and comprise up to eight individuals including alpha parents, young-of-the-year, and their older offspring (Bekoff, 2004). This arrangement works well for the alpha couple and their pups, and to a lesser extent for their offspring helpers. It is difficult or impossible for these young helpers to form packs of their own, so their next best chance of getting their genes into the gene pool is to assist in the raising of their brothers and sisters who share their genetic inheritance. Offspring males stay with the pack as helpers to their parents longer than do females, as evolutionary theory predicts: females know that their young are their own, while males can never be sure that the young born to their partner are actually theirs, too. Male helpers are as certain of their sibling relationship to their mother's offspring as are their sisters. However, if these brother and sister helpers each should have their own progeny, the sister would know her youngsters were hers while the brother could not be sure of the paternity of his.

BEAVER FAMILIES

To sit beside a quiet pond on a fall evening and watch a beaver (*Castor canadensis*) slip through the water toward the dam, another on the bank sorting out aspen branches, and a third chomping lily pads gives the impression that individual beaver lead separate lives. If you watch closely, though, these individuals touch noses or rub faces in greeting when they encounter each other during their forays, even though they all live in the same crowded lodge. Indeed, especially in the north of their range, beaver are surely the most social mammals in the world. What other species has members who spend half the year huddled together in tiny dark quarters, frozen in so completely that their only outlet is to dive into the water and swim under thick ice? Talk about "cabin fever"! They feel their confinement, though; with warm weather, they celebrate their release from the ice with non-stop aquabatics – plunging under and over each other as they speed around the pond, exuberantly rolling and somersaulting in sheer euphoria to be out in the fresh air.

Hope Ryden (1989) observed the activities of members of a beaver family by sitting beside their pond during evenings and nights, year after year. When she first met them in Harriman State Park, 65 km (40 mi) north of New York City, the large 27 kg (60 lb) male she called The Inspector General (because she often saw him inspecting the dam for leaks) was Lily's partner; the pair had two kits whom she named Laurel and Skipper. (Skipper was presumed to be male until she was observed, years later, suckling her own kits. Beaver have a cloaca which encloses their reproductive organs, making it difficult to determine their sex.) The animals were innately good natured. If there was a squabble over food, it was solved by wrestling or shoving against each other, not by a bite from their strong incisors, which could have been lethal. They ate together, groomed themselves or each other, and sometimes played, diving and splashing in the water.

The following spring, Lily produced two kits, Lotus and Blossom, who lived in the lodge for their first month. There is always the danger that a young kit whose fur is not yet waterproof will fall into the underwater entrance and drown, so they are never left alone. Ryden saw both parents and Laurel and Skipper, now adults, taking turns of an evening to haul fresh grass bedding and food into the lodge and remain there with the kits to ensure their safety. When these young were old enough to venture into the pond, adults stayed near them, bringing them food and letting them ride on their backs. Gradually, the kits learned what beaver do by watching their seniors at the different tasks of reinforcing the dam or lodge, cutting down trees, lopping off branches, and hauling them into the water for winter supplies. The kits sometimes swiped food from their siblings just as did their parents, so there seemed to be no dominance hierarchy in the family based on age or sex. The young were obviously a family enterprise.

The Inspector General and Lily willingly allowed all of their older progeny to share their food or the lodge because there were no new territories available in the area for them to occupy. Ryden's family expanded until, in year three, there were eight beaver wintering in the lodge, which measured over a meter (about 4 ft) in diameter. After that the family began to disperse, perhaps in some cases a brother and sister setting up a new family for lack of fresh blood. These new pairs were not formed because of the urge to reproduce. They got together in the summer or fall, although they would not mate and start a family until about February; it was essential for them to build a lodge together and store food in order to survive the winter. Then they, too, could look forward to a satisfactory life enjoyed with their yearly litters. Incest is rare in animals, but most likely in species such as beaver who have a heavy investment in their territory and the dam and house they have built. As an analogy, some very rich people who want to keep their wealth within the family are known to foster cousin marriages for their children.

Recent research sheds light on activity in a beaver lodge using four new techniques pioneered by Donald Griffin: direct observation and filming from a blind attached to a lodge, continuous recording with microphones, radiotelemetry, and videorecording by means of a spy camera inserted into the lodge (Müller-Schwarze and Sun, 2003). However, in winter there is little more to see than beaver dragging in food, eating it, and snoozing. There is no possibility of seeing if two beaver in the squeeze of fur and flesh are special friends. At this time, beaver are so disconnected from the outside world that recordings of their periodic gnawing sounds reveal that their summer 24-hour day of activities has turned into a 26.5-hour day.

Beaver have an excellent sense of smell related to the castoreum scent that they place on mounds around their territory to alert other beaver that their pond or river area is taken. It enables individuals to recognize their relations from their smell, even if they have never met. Dietland Müller-Schwarze and Lixing Sun (2003), in their research on beaver in the Allegany State Park, New York, discovered this when a young beaver, leaving his natal pond, moved two kilometers (1.2 mi) downstream and stayed for two months with his grandparents, whom he had never met, before moving on to make a new life elsewhere. Had they not been related, the grandparents would have attacked him instead of making him welcome.

CROW FAMILIES

American crows (*Corvus brachyrhynchos*) often form family groups that are closely bonded for long periods of time. Like most birds who produce poorly developed altricial nestlings, there is a close bond between breeding males and females as they raise their young. They both work long hours to bring enough food for their rapid growth. But do crows migrate and return to their natal area in future years? Does the mating-bond last from one year to the next? Do older progeny team up with their parents to help raise the next generation? To answer such questions, birds must be marked individually in some way.

To this end, graduate student John Withey and his supervisor, John Marzluff of the University of Washington's College of Forest Resources in Seattle, perfected a tiny radio transmitter that weighed about 3 percent of a crow's body weight, to be fastened onto a crow's back with a harness of teflon ribbon (Marzluff and Angell, 2005). The device ran on a single battery that lasted for up to two years. To band the legs of individual crows and attach these transmitters to the backs of many of them, the men had first to trap them. This was a challenge.

Trapping birds is difficult, but trapping crows is a nightmare. First, the men heaped white bread near a hidden net camouflaged with vegetation. When crows walked up to this tasty treat, a net triggered by a gun flew out of the bushes and over them with a loud bang, so that they were trapped. This worked initially, but any crow who witnessed this horror remembered it for a year or more. A third of them never again approached the bread or the net. Those who did, took an average of 43 long minutes to inch toward the food supply, with "sidestepping, staring, overflights and aborted tries." That many minutes per bird is a lot of time to wait to launch the net while cooped up in a blind. The crows also remembered the men who had put them through the indignity of being prodded, poked, measured, and banded. When the two researchers walked across the university campus among hundreds of students and faculty, crows who had been caught and banded recognized them and called repeatedly so that their fellows would know that the evil trappers were at large.[4]

With many birds finally banded, the researchers were able to prove that crows do indeed mate for life. Such pairs paid close attention to each other throughout the year: perching side by side, flying or walking together, calling softly, gently touching bills, or preening. To allopreen, whether on a wire, in a tree, or on the ground, one crow (usually the female) edged up to her partner, nodded briefly, and raised her head feathers. The partner then deftly picked through the feathers with his beak to remove any dirt or parasites from hard-to-reach areas. There has to be great trust between the couple to allow the strong beak of one so close to the other's head and eyes, so this activity undoubtedly strengthened their pair-bond.

Even when they were bonded, the male still courted the female, flying high above her and giving acrobatic dives and rolls to display his skill. She showed her readiness to mate by crouching down with her wings held out and drooping, her tail vibrating up and down. The male might take this position too. When the eggs were laid, he often brought the female food, transferring it from his bill to hers as she sat on the nest; with food supplied, she could spend more time covering the eggs to keep them warm and perhaps increase the clutch size. Together the pair fed their hatched youngsters a wide variety of food, from vegetation to insects to scavenged meat to baby birds; studies have counted 650 different food items in crow stomachs.

Helpers to the breeding pair of crows form an important part of many crow families, both in this species and in other related corvids. In his study of American crows in Florida, Lawrence Kilham (1989) actually found that *all* the breeding pairs had helpers, so there were no controls for him to compare and estimate how effective such auxiliaries were in the production of healthy young. Helper numbers are higher where there are few or no territories without breeding crows nearby. This may explain why family size was greater in urban (about five per family) than in rural habitats, where they might be shot (about three per family), in Massachusetts. Helpers are usually siblings to the new brood, although some may be unrelated to the parents. They were not of much use to the breeding pair for territorial defence – they cawed from a distance rather than getting actively involved in any altercation – but they were useful in locating food and detecting possible danger. Many also helped in familial tasks, such as building the nest where the female would lay her eggs by carrying sticks and lumps of mud and turf to the nest site. When the eggs hatched, they brought food to the nestlings. All such activity was a learning curve for the young which who would help them when they themselves became breeding birds a year or two later. (Kilham also noticed a down-side to helpers; sometimes they interfered with nest construction or interrupted copulations and incubation. Rarely, a female helper tried to seduce the breeding male.)

Crows may collect in large congregations in winter. In Ontario, many hundreds often assemble in trees at a different location each night – one such noisy mass gathering occurred outside my window in a cold January – so individuals must communicate daily somehow to set up these conventions. Related to this ability to organize is surely the large size of the corvid brain which, compared to body size, is about as complex as that of apes (Woolfson, 2008). As we have seen for many social primates, evolution of increasing brain size and complexity correlates with extensive interactions between individuals.

GIBBON GROUPS

We have seen in the chapter: *Male and female pals – not just for sex!* that gibbon male and female adult pairs usually raise young together over a number of years. A young male, as he reaches full size at about eight years of age, has four options for his future (Brockelman *et al.*, 1998):

(a)   challenge and defeat a territorial male so he can take over the territory and start his own family,

(b)   compete for and fill the vacancy left by the death of a territory holder,

(c)   inherit or cut off a portion of the parental territory for his own use, or

(d)   remain in the natal territory for an extra few years, benefiting the family with grooming, social play with the young who often lack a playmate, and support of their father in defending the territory. This multigenerational family gets along well, eating at fruiting trees, playing, resting, and sleeping. They seem the best of friends.

Gibbons do not necessarily live in nuclear families as was once assumed, but often have more complex relationships bonded together. Warren Brockelman and his colleagues (1998) calculated that if a gibbon group contained two young less than two years apart in age (because the minimum birth interval for a female is three years), then these two could not be siblings and therefore did not live in a nuclear family. From a census of 64 gibbon groups (*Hylobates lar*) in a Thailand forest, one-third of them contained young who were less than two years apart in age. Indeed, of the groups that the researchers had observed intensely, most of them comprised non-nuclear relationships, including half-siblings, nieces, nephews, and even unrelated individuals. They describe one such group of gibbons after the resident male had been displaced; it comprised a young juvenile presumably fathered by the ousted resident male, two younger juveniles (probably brothers) from the new male's original group and, later, offspring of the new pair. Members of this group got along well, the adults grooming all the young and all the young playing together.

Other species in close groups

This section features five species' groups with unusual affinities. Woolly spider monkeys have close bonds within either sex; black-handed spider monkey males are friendly among themselves but the females are inclined to be loners; lesser kudu have buddies among the females but not the males; white rhinoceros hook up with one or two other individuals for fairly short-term alliances; and sperm whales remain something of an enigma. These as well as other species have not been studied extensively or in a variety of habitats, so further research may modify our ideas about their behaviors.

WOOLLY SPIDER MONKEYS OR MURIQUIS

For woolly spider monkeys (*Brachyteles arachnoides*), where the members of each sex are tightly bonded and non-aggressive, groups can seem like small love-ins. When the animals are resting, 65 percent of the time they are within a one meter (1 yd) radius of each other, although they spread out more when they are feeding (Strier, 1992). If one individual feels friendly, he or she indicates this with a light touch to the body or a full-bodied (literally) embrace of another, during which the two animals hang by their long prehensile tails with their arms and legs wrapped around each other. Embraces usually occur when the individuals are moving about between resting or feeding sites, during or following a threat to a group from another group, or when a male wants to check whether a female is nearing estrus.

Adult females were most likely to embrace in dyads (42 percent of all embraces seen). However, because almost all females emigrate to another troop just before they reach puberty, the females in this population all ended up in the Jaò troop, the only other one within reach, which presumably would not have happened in the past when woolly spider monkey numbers were greater. Therefore, in this study, at least, they kept their close ties with their sisters and with early female friends who had also emigrated. The possibility of inbreeding was much higher than normal with only two troops in the area, but Strier did not know if there was a troop taboo against incest.

The second most common dyad combination to embrace were adult males and females (25 percent of all embraces seen); these were often related to mating, but in one case a mother and her adult son enjoyed a leisurely hug (see the chapter: *Mothers and sons, and providing free food*). There is no jealousy about copulations. If males and females do not socialize on a daily basis, estrus females will spread their urine by hand on branches and leaves to alert passing males to their reproductive condition. These females openly accept lengthy mountings from males; when one copulation is complete, they turn to another male who has been patiently waiting his turn. Rivalry between males has been replaced by sperm competition among mating males. A copulatory plug begins to form in a female's vagina after each copulation, but she or a male may pluck it out and eat it before it can harden.

Rather than embrace in pairs, adult males tend to form an intense embracing huddle in which they not only confirm their solidarity, but also assess each other's hug-strength. It was difficult for Strier to figure out whether embraces were equated with social bonds because, for example, although 37 percent of Scruff's embraces were with Nancy, he otherwise only spent one percent of his time in close proximity to her. Among males, though, embrace rates were positively correlated to the proportion of time the males spent close together during resting, while males that associated closely with each other tended also to interact most often (Strier *et al.*, 2002).

Members of Strier's Matão group kept close track of each other by exchanging a variety of neighs, chuckles, warbles, and chirps that conveyed such emotions as reassurance, excitement, or quiet companionship. The loud neighs served to keep the group in contact in dense vegetation, each monkey producing his or her own distinctive call. Soft chirps while feeding seemed rather like pleasant chat carried on among people working together. All the vocalizations also served to keep the other troop away, and so prevent fighting over sources of fruit.

BLACK-HANDED SPIDER MONKEYS

Most people visit Tikal National Park in Guatemala to admire the marvellous pyramids and ruins of an ancient Mayan city, but Linda Marie Fedigan and Margaret Joan Baxter (1984) came for six months to watch the activities of black-handed spider monkeys (*Ateles geoffroyi*) who live there. Because the area is an extensive archeological site, many well-mapped trails criss-cross the forest floor, enabling an observer to keep up with a troop moving through the foliage overhead. If a human follower were bothersome, a monkey above might shake a branch or give an open-mouth expression of annoyance, but in general they were well habituated to humans and protected in the park from hunting and poaching. Focal sessions for observing each individual were only five minutes long because it was hard to keep arboreal animals moving fast in sight. The troops were large, of perhaps 75 monkeys, so it was difficult to recognize the individuals. The researchers therefore analyzed their data by age and sex (although the males and females were about the same size), recording these categories along with the 33 behaviors that the monkeys exhibited.

The researchers did not recognize the monkeys individually, so it is impossible to know if there were some pairs who preferred being together more than other duos. They did find a large amount of social activity among the males, but much less among the females. The males and females kept to themselves when they foraged and traveled, the males in groups and the females alone or with their offspring. They only came together to rest, play, and sleep at night. Although the females were often alone or dispersed, they did keep in touch while feeding with soft vocal calls, and did occasionally spend time with other monkeys. Most multimale groups of primates exhibit high levels of aggression, but this was not true for the black-handed spider monkeys. Rather than fighting among themselves, the males form into cohesive units. They embraced, sat in contact with each other, and directed "the vast majority of their affinitive behaviors" to other males and their aggressive behaviors to females (who did not reciprocate) and to members of rival groups.

Kathy Slater and two colleagues (2009) recently carried out research, over 17 months, on this same species of spider monkey in Yucatan, Mexico. Their subjects belonged to two groups, both smaller than those at Tikal. They defined a new affirmative behavior, arm wrapping, where two individuals wrapped their arms around the other's neck, both facing the same direction, in an aggressive coalition against people or other animals. Although interactions among animals were infrequent, they resembled those at Tikal, with relationships between males of high quality, those between females of low quality, and those of mixed sexes unsettling, with males harassing females with threats, chases, lunges, strikes, and bites. Such aggression never occurred between the six known mother–adult son dyads, though. When males were in a mixed-sex group, they embraced each other more than usual, as if to reduce the likelihood of aggression where males might compete for mating rights. Females did embrace new mothers so they could have access to their infants – most species value their young.

LESSER KUDU

Lesser kudu (*Tragelaphus imberbis*) are medium-sized antelope who live in small groups in dense scrub and semi-arid bush country in Africa. They are brown with white vertical body stripes in individualized patterns, which allowed Walter Leuthold (1974) to name and recognize 95 adults. He made cards for each, with photographs or sketches of their coat markings so that a spotter with binoculars, standing on a seat of a landrover and looking through the roof hatch, could recognize individuals as the vehicle cruised along roads in the Tsavo National Park in Kenya. Each week over a period of several years, the vehicle covered about 650 km (400 mi). It was tricky work, because when the landrover was in motion, the lesser kudu would allow it to drive within 20 or 30 meters (about 80 ft) of them, but when it stopped, they immediately fled into the bush. Leuthold made notes of the individuals he could see, but often was unable to recognize all of them if there were more than one or two. In addition, he noted the sex and size of each animal along with the horn shape of the males.

The lesser kudu had small home ranges where they were often sighted, but seldom in very large numbers. Usually just a few hung out together; for instance, several females and their young, if any. For example, female 2, who was seen a total of 27 times, was sighted most often with females 3 and 6. Female 3 was noted at 16 of these sightings, and possibly five more times when she may have been present but not recognized. Of a total of 20 occasions, female 6 was seen with female 2 ten times, and she could have been present eight other times but not recognized. Groups that included female 2 numbered from one to nine, so other animals were sometimes present as well. Leuthold concluded that females 2, 3, and 6 in effect formed a stable nuclear group whose friendship lasted over at least eight months. Other females joined this group now and then and sometimes an adult male did so, although most adult males kept to themselves. There were, therefore, no similar friendships among the males, nor between males and females.

WHITE RHINOCEROS

White rhinoceros (*Ceratotherium simum*) are more social than black rhinoceros, hanging out usually in a group. Adrian Shrader and Norman Owen-Smith (2002) decided to carry out research on how these animals disperse from the area where they were born, leading to a possible later extension of their (or even their species') range. They discovered that those rhinoceros who made excursions outside their home range did so with one or more companions, referred to as a "buddy system." These exploring animals were of either sex, at least five years of age up to the age of socio-sexual maturity (about seven years for females and eleven for males), and their associates were either a friend of similar age or an adult female without a calf. They had all been living apart from their mother since they were two or three years old, chased away by her after she produced her next offspring.

Dispersing into unknown territory is a risky business, whether through pressure from other rhinoceros to leave or the urge to find new resources of food and water. By doing so with a friend or two, a rhinoceros reduces the chance of being attacked by lions or territorial rhinoceros males and becomes familiar with a new habitat, especially if he or she is guided by a companion more familiar with this new area. Such companions were often from an overlapping home range.

The scientists carried out their research in the Hluhluwe–Umfolozi Park in South Africa, over a two-year period, where there was a population of about 1600 white rhinoceros. Small radio transmitters were inserted into the front horn of newly adult rhinoceros (five males and two females) so that their travels and their companions could be monitored; a few other rhinoceros were observed closely as well. The home ranges of these individuals were established over many months by GPS (global positioning system) equipment so that their excursions into new territories could be identified. These excursions, which lasted a day or two, were as long as 12 km (7.5 mi). Associations between animals who hung out together and at some point made such excursions could last for up to five months or more.

Detailed results showed that all seven of the monitored animals made at least one excursion outside their home range, for a total of 20 in all. About one-quarter of the excursions were made with another young adult who had been a stable companion for some time, another quarter with a long-term adult female friend, and the remaining half with individuals who had been companions for less than a month or even just for the length of the excursion. Many excursions were with a single friend, sometimes two friends together made several excursions, and some excursions involved up to five animals.

In an earlier paper, Norman Owen-Smith (1974) noted that sometimes two cows, each without calves, and perhaps in some cases a mother and her adult daughter, join forces. He reports that females are so socially minded that they will usually accept the company of others, with the result that solitary cows are rarely seen.

SPERM WHALES

Sperm whales (*Physeter macrocephalus*) have stable female groups because four pairs of females who had metal tags shot into their blubber, in the North Pacific, were still together hundreds of kilometers distant when they were killed, and the tags recovered between five and ten years later (Whitehead, 2003). This does not mean that they were together as a pair, though, but only that both belonged to the same permanent group. Sperm whale expert Hal Whitehead of Dalhousie University in Halifax, Nova Scotia, who has analyzed the basic social units of sperm whales, decided that, in the big picture, females do not have particular friends, but rather together form a permanent group with homogenous bonds between all the members. At any one time, the sperm whales whom one may be lucky enough to see swimming in the ocean comprise perhaps one permanent social unit, whose members (females, subadult males, and young – Whitehead calls them "constant companions") may or may not be related to each other. Some individuals may be "casual acquaintances" who remain with the group for only a few hours or days. The permanent members of a unit all hang out together, swimming, resting, feeding, vocalizing, leaping into the air, and often rubbing against each other (Gordon, 1998). (All whales and dolphins have sensitive skin, which they like to have touched or rubbed.) When a mother dives deep for squid, her newborn young cannot follow her, so it is protected on the surface by other females; grandmothers who continue to lactate after they are too old themselves to reproduce suckle such infants (Whitehead, 2003). Two social units of whales may swim along together for several days but then they separate again. That no whales within a unit were more likely to swim beside one individual rather than another surprised Whitehead. He therefore speculated that because the animals do not compete for food, which is found in huge areas in the deep ocean, no issues of inequity would occur between them. Therefore, there would be little advantage in forming specific partnerships. Non-breeding male sperm whales form their own loose groups that spend much of their time in the subarctic where food is abundant.

In summary, a few mammals have groups so closely bonded that the members are in close contact with each other every day of their lives. Smaller family groups may share such friendship too. White rhinoceros hang out together and may join a friend or friends to seek out new territories and, as far as we know, sperm whales may too.

As animals age, some are no longer interested in sex. They become less active within their community, but often still value a friend with whom to be companionable, as we shall see in the following chapter.

Old buddies

By the time an animal is old, often he or she is no longer reproducing or following the customs of their youth. They are free spirits
who may team up with another chum to spend their last days in
congenial company. This has been documented for mountain gorillas,
olive baboons, gelada baboons, elephants, African buffalo, and red
deer. A final short section on loners identifies single animals who
seem to want company.

MOUNTAIN GORILLAS

Dian Fossey (1983) only encountered Rafiki and Coco when they
were old, their group without youngsters, so it is perhaps the
lack of preadolescents needing protection that made the group so
easy to habituate to her presence. Rafiki was about fifty years old, a
usually tolerant silverback leader of group 8 which comprised, as
well as himself, a young silverback (Pug), a blackback in his prime
(Samson), two young males (Geezer and Peanut), and a serene but
decrepit old female with light coat color (Coco). Fossey named the
leader Rafiki, which means "friend" in Swahili, because friendship implied the mutual trust and respect she felt for him. She
believed that Coco was the mother of Samson and Peanut who
resembled her.

Rafiki and Coco acted like an old married couple, together most
of the day and often sleeping in the same nest. Coco was not given to
moving about much, but she often initiated mutual grooming sessions
with the males, picking through their fur to remove bits of dry skin and
parasites. The males were always solicitous of her, despite her wrinkled
face, balding head and rump, graying muzzle, flabby upper arms,
missing teeth, and failing sight and hearing. Sometimes she sat

hunched over by herself, one arm crossed over her chest and the other rapidly patting the top of her head.

One of Fossey's fondest early memories of the gorillas was a scenario of the wonderful rapport between Rafiki and Coco she witnessed while in hiding. Group 8 was feeding on an open hillside. Coco was below the others, hunting for leaves to eat and wandering uncertainly away from the rest of the group. Rafiki, who was above her, suddenly glanced down and gave a call, at which she stopped and turned to go toward the sound. Rafiki and the others sat down as if to wait for her. Coco slowly worked her way up the hill, stopping now and then to see where they might be, until she spotted Rafiki and moved directly toward him, giving a series of soft noises. When she reached him, they looked into each other's eyes and embraced. He put his arm around her shoulders and she did the same to him as they carried on slowly up the hill, murmuring together. The younger troop members slowly followed them, feeding along the way, until they all went over the hill where Fossey could no longer see them.

Soon, because Coco was becoming too weak to keep up with the group, Rafiki began to shorten their travel routes to suit her. One February day in 1968 when Fossey arrived at group 8, Rafiki and Coco were no longer there with the four younger males. Backtracking along the trail of the group, she found that the two gorillas had slept in the same nest for the past two nights, but then all trace of them had disappeared. Rafiki came back to the group two days later, but Coco was never seen again, and was presumed dead. Their close bond was broken.

Old Rafiki lived for another seven years. With Coco no longer present, the five males of group 8 began to squabble among themselves. The two males whom Coco had not borne left the group, and Rafiki quarreled especially with his elder son, Samson, as noted in the chapter: *Fathers and sons, and social grooming and preening*. Two years after Coco's death, Maisie and Macho joined Rafiki, causing further confrontations between him and Samson, who wanted females of his own. He also left the group until two years later, when he had his revenge by coming back and persuading Maisie to go away with him. They had a son in 1972, and Rafiki and Macho a daughter a year later. After a full life, Rafiki died in 1974 of pneumonia and pleurisy.

OLIVE BABOONS

Boz and Alexander were elderly buddies, as Barbara Smuts (1985) describes in her book *Sex and Friendship in Baboons* about olive baboons living in the Great Rift Valley of Kenya. As we saw in the chapter: *Male and female pals – not just for sex!*, special friendships between adult males and females are a central feature of baboon society – indeed, Alexander had a good thing going with the female Thalia, and Boz with six females including Iolanthe – Smuts describes Iolanthe rushing to meet Boz who was returning from a trip; he gently touched the infant on her back before he walked with her, side by side, to rejoin the other baboons.

However, Boz was especially devoted to Alexander. As the elder, he sometimes defended him when there was a fight. Once, when Boz heard Alexander scream some distance away because he was being attacked by another male, he rushed to his rescue, leaping on the back of the assailant. Every morning when the pair woke up, they sought each other out for a ritual greeting. This could be of three types, all brief, and all practiced to some extent by all the males, even though the prime animals usually thought of each other as rivals. Each greeting began when one male, X, usually the more dominant, approached another, Y, with a swinging gait, often lip-smacking while staring into Y's eyes. If Y returned the stare, often lip-smacking as well, the greeting continued with Y either using a hip grasp on X, diddling X's genitals, or mounting X. If either broke off the ritualized sequence by turning aside, the greeting was aborted.

Barbara Smuts and John Watanabe (1990), who observed this male greeting 637 times during 93 hours of observation, found that in a number of ways Alexander and Boz had a closer relationship than did other dyads. They greeted each other much more often than most pairs; the greeting involved mounting behavior (seldom seen between prime males) more often than hip-grasping or diddling; almost all of their greeting ceremonies were completed (unlike greetings between two prime males, which were often broken off); they used genital diddling more often than others, which is the most risky and intimate form of contact; and, most strikingly, they were the only ones to show complete symmetry in their active and passive roles. If one was a mounter on one occasion, the other would be at their next greeting; the same thing happened with diddling and hip grasping. Alexander and Boz also teamed up with each other to lure estrus females away from younger prime males so they could mate with them; each was too old to defeat a younger male by himself.

This tender story of Alexander and Boz is atypical, though. Robert Sapolsky (1996), who has spent nearly 30 years studying baboon behavior in East Africa, notes that, in general, "Male baboons do not have male friends. I can count on one hand the number of times I've seen adult males grooming one another over the years." They may join together to form a "business" coalition, but this is a short-term, uneasy partnership at best. They often, of course, have female Friends as we saw in the chapter: *Male and female pals – not just for sex!* Those males who have eschewed such friendships often leave the troop when they reach old age because of aggression and lack of member support. Those who have developed companionship with females and become a part of the community over the years tend to spend their final years "still mating, grooming, being groomed, sitting in contact with females, interacting with infants." Friendship can make the difference between a serene old age and one of dispossession.

Leah and Gums were two old olive baboons esteemed by Robert Sapolsky (2001), who denoted Gums as a nondescript male of "vast decrepitude" and "ancient Leah" as the female who had spent much of her lifetime harassing her social inferior Naomi. Sapolsky was appalled one morning to find that these two oldest baboons had vanished from the troop on the same day. He wondered if hyenas or a leopard could have killed and eaten them. Ten days later, he was thrilled to see them sitting side by side in the distance while he was driving through an area he seldom visited. They gave a start when they noticed his vehicle and, although they had been used to people snooping around their troop for years, they now reacted with panic, Leah loping off into a thicket, followed by Gums. The next day, Sapolsky drove by the same site again and, in the distance, observed them resting together in a field of wildflowers. He never saw them after that, but obviously they had decided to spend their last days together.

GELADA BABOONS

Gelada baboons (*Theropithecus gelada gelada*) of Ethiopia congregate in the largest groups of any primate, numbering as many as 350 animals who spend most of their time foraging on grass and herbs. One major component of a troop are the family units each comprising one breeding alpha male (plus maybe one or two non-breeding males), about three (one to eight) adult females in a dominance hierarchy, and their young (Ohsawa, 1979). These animals are constantly in touch, either near each other physically or calling aloud to maintain contact. The male and females get along fairly well, with grooming now and then, although the alpha female may try to keep the other females away from the male boss (Mori, 1979b).

The other major component of a troop are the loose all-male units comprising a few males of various ages, whose adult members tend to pick fights with an alpha male to try to take over his family unit (Mori, 1979c). There is no friendly behavior between members of different units (Mori, 1979a).

The third minor grouping which interests us here is of bonded pairs, which include an old female who is no longer reproducing and, unlike the younger females, no longer under the control of an alpha male (Ohsawa, 1979). One pair was the male Brown and the female Kireme in K-herd; another such couple lived in A-herd. Such pairs forage where they want without reference to other units. Another pair, Fukunyu and Nimesu, were two fairly old females with the K-herd, again with no offspring in sight; they were attacked repeatedly by other members of the K-herd and eventually disappeared. Young and prime females who were kept in check by their unit males were never seen in pairs. It is pleasant to imagine old unrestrained females at last having a special pal with whom they can relax to do whatever they want.

ELEPHANTS

Very old male elephants sometimes team up with a younger bull near rivers, where there is soft vegetation that the elder is able to eat with his worn teeth. This younger male may act as a guard, or even help his friend pull down branches for food. Sylvia Sikes (1971) surmised that this chum might be sexually non-functional for some reason or unable to hold his own in a male herd, but he was surely a comrade keeping company with his old buddy. She notes from personal observation that such attendant bulls often had injuries such as paralysis of the trunk, lameness, broken tusks, blindness, or lop-ears, which might explain why they had retired from active bull herds. Sikes writes that "Nature is never 'kind' in the human sense," although she herself, in the 1960s, hunted and killed many elephants, destroying the heart and integrity of their families in the process; she did this under the auspices of the British Heart Foundation and Zoological Society of London so that she could examine their hearts and other organs.

AFRICAN BUFFALO

The African buffalo (*Syncerus caffer*) is considered one of the fiercest animals in Africa, willing to attack without cause any human being on foot, but when a male grows old, he gives up his aggressive ways and often leaves his large mixed-sex herd to become close chums with another buffalo. Are they tired of the hurly-burly of large groups? Or no longer interested in mating? Or can they no longer keep up with their younger associates? We do not know. Many authors have seen such elderly pairs who are no longer a menace to them.

Dian Fossey (1983) was pleased to have two old buffalo friends living near her cabin at Karisoke, the research base for her study of gorillas. They chose this area perhaps because Fossey kept it as a refuge free from poachers. The male she called Mzee, the Swahili name for an old man. His hide was criss-crossed with scars from past encounters with poachers, traps, and other buffalo over his long life; his horns were worn down to mere nubbins. With him was an old female, who slowly led the way along mountain paths, as if aware of his failing eyesight. This was odd for a female, because although most old male buffalo leave their herd in old age, elderly females usually remain with their group.

Daphne Sheldrick (1973) reports two such couples in her book *Animal Kingdom: The Story of Tsavo, the Great African Game Park*. Her husband, the Park Game Warden, noted a buffalo standing beside a pile of bleached bones on one occasion, but thought no more about it. On a later flight, seeing the same odd sight, he dived low in his airplane. The animal refused to be driven away from the bones; instead, he tossed his head and pawed the ground as if to defend the remains of his long-dead companion. Sheldrick comments that most people who kill an animal do not give a thought for the sorrow and misery their action causes his or her friends.

Mark Mloszewski (1983) observed two old, strongly bonded, bachelor buffalo in Kenya. One who was blind and probably deaf was helped by his buddy, who always rubbed against him before moving away so that the other would know it was time to go. The two then walked along together until it was time to halt, at which point the buddy blocked the way of his impaired mate to physically stop him. The two then grazed, or rested, or drank, as was appropriate. If the impaired bull sensed an emergency, he stood at the alert, waiting for the other to push against him to indicate in which direction they should flee. If only his healthy partner perceived danger, he would make body contact with his blind companion before rushing off. He apparently was able to signal information about the peril in this way.

Dick Pitman (2007) described two old bull buffalo lolling in mud on the river bank while he was boating in Zimbabwe. The two oldsters

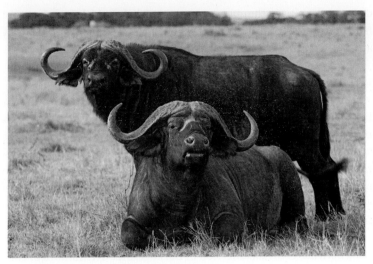

Figure 8. African buffalo – old buddies.
© photolibrary.com

heaved themselves wearily onto their feet when they saw the boat, in case they should feel the need to retreat from the craft.

Mark and Delia Owens (2006) first nervously welcomed an old buffalo pair to their wilderness camp in Zambia's North Luangwa National Park on the Luangwa River because of their size and the species' reputation. When the Owens had initially moved there in 1986, buffalo were too wary to come close because so many had been massacred by poachers. They stayed in thickets on the far side of the river, even after they could see that puku antelope, warthogs, and elephants felt secure enough to roam among the park huts. After years, several ventured into the camp under cover of darkness to graze. Later they spent the night in the long grass by the river before wandering slowly toward the camp each morning, watching with interest people walking about. First Brutus arrived, who scared Delia badly when she nearly bumped into him on a path in the dark. Then came his friend Bad-Ass, an equally large male who had the discomfiting habit of lowering his head and hooking the air with his horns. Later another old buffalo pair joined them: Stubby who had a stub of a tail and Nubbin whose horns were worn down. The locals named the four the Kakule Club, the ChiBemba word for old male buffalo. Eventually they felt so at home in the camp, where they were safe from lions and poachers, that they spent entire days grazing, resting, chewing their cud, and sleeping in the open area near the kitchen. Male buffalo do not hang out together for any period when they are in their prime, but they are happy to do so when they have become elders.

RED DEER

In his book *A Herd of Red Deer*, Fraser Darling (1969) notes that during his research in Scotland, in summer it was fairly common to see an old stag (*Cervus elaphus*) along with one or two young males, who kept themselves clear of the other deer. He describes, watching through binoculars, an old ten-point stag and a young one lying down near each other about 400 yards (365 m) away. Suddenly, the young male spotted Darling and froze, the cud he had been chewing motionless in his mouth. He got up, trotted over to the old stag, and lowered his muzzle to his friend's face. They both stared in the direction of Darling. After five minutes of complete stillness by both Darling and the stags, the animals relaxed. The youngster moved away, lay down, and again began to chew his cud. The old stag lowered his head and closed his eyes. Ten minutes later, Darling moved again, this time onto his knees. Again the young male spotted the motion and trotted to the old stag. This time, the oldster struggled to his feet while they both gazed intently in Darling's direction for five more minutes. Then they grazed perfunctorily, lay down again, and relaxed. At this time red deer were hunted in the area, which explains the wariness of the two friends. Soon Darling crept away to leave them in peace.

LONERS

Often an old male from a social species is alone, probably because he has no one with whom to associate. Delia and Mark Owens (2006) describe meeting single old lions in the Kalahari Desert who wandered about by themselves, sometimes standing on a termite mound staring into the distance for minutes at a time, "'cooing' into the wind, inviting social contact among pride-mates who were no longer there to hear them." When two old males chanced to meet, even if they had not been pride-mates, they would hang out together for companionship. The Owens sometimes encountered lone bull wildebeest in the Kalahari too, who would follow their landrover whenever it came near them; it seemed that even a vehicle was company of some sort.

This chapter indicates that members of social species, especially males, as they grow old may leave a group to associate with one other individual. Because they are no longer involved in mating or in raising young, they can opt out of community life and the rigors of reproducing or trying to do so (for males), and relax to enjoy golden months with a companion.

Some social species comprise members who always move about in groups but who have no interest in each other; individuals hang out together largely for protection against predators. They usually do the same things at the same time, feeding, traveling, and resting, but forming friendly dyads within their group is not in their repertoire, as we shall see in the following chapter.

Social but seldom sociable animals

Some species are social in that they live in groups, but the animals within the groups are not friendly with each other. This chapter will deal with three categories which include species of this nature: primates, large herbivores, and meerkats.

Primates

Primates considered in this chapter are squirrel monkeys, colobine monkeys, patas monkeys, hamadryas baboons, and sifaka lemurs. Some theorists postulate that the evolution of friendships among female primates depends, to a large extent, upon the environment, especially the food they eat, as we shall see in the discussion of squirrel monkeys. Lynne Isbell and Truman Young (2002) hypothesize on the significance of food and other factors in the life of primates:

(a) Accessibility of food: In species that eat high-quality food growing in clumps, females should be philopatric (remain in their natal area for life) and defend the food source aggressively against members of other groups. In areas with food uniformly distributed or in small high-quality clumps, the females should emigrate at puberty, lack dominance hierarchies, and not quarrel with other groups given that their food source is not really defensible.

(b) Dominance hierarchy: Food that is spread out and largely indefensible can still be problematic. There can be scramble competition for it, meaning that the individuals who get to it first will reduce it for others by eating it themselves, and contest competition whereby high-ranking individuals showing aggression can gain preferential access to the food.

(c) Relationships: If females in a group are closely related, they should support each other (nepotism) in order to increase the number of their joint progeny.

(d) Possibility of infanticide: If members of a species sometimes kill the offspring of females, then these females should bond together to try to prevent this catastrophe.

(e) Heavy predation: If a species is subject to intense predation, the females might band together to counter-attack (depending on the size of the predator) and/or prefer to stay close together to try to detect the danger and evade it.

In contrast to this environmental theory for female behavior, male behavior is largely driven by their instinctual wish to be near females, so that they can detect those who are in estrus and mate with as many of them as are willing.

SQUIRREL MONKEYS

Research into different species of squirrel monkeys in South and Central America illustrates how the previously described factors interact and how, even though the little creatures do not spend all that much time filling their small stomachs, their food sources can critically shape their behavior. Carol Mitchell and two colleagues (1991) compared the lives of *Saimiri oerstedii* and *S. sciureus*, monkeys scarcely larger than squirrels who are at high risk of predation. Both live in large groups, presumably to improve the detection of, and create confusion for, such predators as raptors, snakes, and ocelots. About three or four *S. oerstedii* fed typically on uniform small patches of fruits while groups of 17 to 18 *S. sciureus* fed on fruit patches that were fairly large and variable. Because of the concentration of their food source, there was a great deal of squabbling among *S. sciureus*, with over 70 times as many aggressive events per hour as in *S. oerstedii*. Related to this belligerence, *S. sciureus* females had linear dominance hierarchies and often coalitions composed of relatives; in addition, when they became adults they chose to stay in their natal group where food was plentiful and defensible. The researchers did not state that the females bonded, though. By contrast, *S. oerstedii* females did not have dominance hierarchies, did not form coalitions of individuals, and they might or might not leave their group when mature to join another. For this species, the absence of competition for food and the dispersal of females when feeding were correlated with "negligible female bonding."

A second paper on the same subject but adding a third squirrel monkey species from Peru to the mix, *S. boliviensis*, corroborated these findings (Boinski *et al.*, 2002). This third species fits, as far as environmental and behavioral characteristics were concerned, between those of the two species in the original study, but nearer to *S. sciureus*. *S. boliviensis* had nearly as many bouts of aggression as *S. sciureus*, and like this species, had a female dominance hierarchy and kin-based female coalitions. However, they also had dense food patches, which correlated with females who competed for food, formed bonds, and stayed in their group when mature.

Can we extract female friendships from such data? Not really. Female *S. oerstedii*, who forage for food that is spread out, do not have female friendships. Females of *S. sciureus* and *S. boliviensis* both fight over food resources, have linear dominance hierarchies, and sometimes kin-based female coalitions, but only in the latter species were female friendships possible. However, the focus of the two papers is not upon friendship per se, and there is no information on individual animals.

COLOBINE MONKEYS

Theoretically, as indicated previously, if females of a species eat foods that are spread out in the environment so that they are readily accessible and cannot be cornered by any one individual or group, these females will not be especially friendly toward each other and will not form alliances. Amanda Korstjens and two colleagues (2002) decided to test this hypothesis by studying the eating behavior of western red colobus monkeys (*Procolobus badius badius*) and western black-and-white colobus monkeys (*Colobus polykomos polykomos*), both species living in the forested Taï National Park in Ivory Coast. Both of these species eat fruit, flowers, and leaves (a foli-frugivore diet), but the species they favored in their foraging overlapped only slightly. The food of the red colobus monkeys was evenly distributed and relatively abundant in the park, while that of the black-and-white colobus monkeys was relatively more clumped.

The researchers found that, in both species, females were not especially friendly to each other, presumably (according to the hypothesis) because food was fairly easy to obtain and could not be controlled. There was a difference, though, that agreed with the hypothesis, in that there was more fighting when the food sources were more clumped. Whereas among the red colobus females aggressive interactions, such as pushing, threatening, biting, hitting, chasing, or stealing another's food, were rare (0.19 interactions per focal observation hour), those among the black-and-white colobus females were three times as common.

Thomas Struhsaker (1975) studied a different subspecies of the red colobus monkey (*Colobus badius tephrosceles*) for over three years in the Kibale Forest Reserve of Uganda, but not only their eating habits. These animals were so difficult to observe that it was impossible to know unequivocally if there were special friendships among them or not. They lived in groups of from 12 to 80 individuals, each with at least two males and a greater number of females and young. For the larger groups or when two neighboring groups mixed together, it was impossible to count the numbers high up in trees in the rain forest, let alone identify various individuals. In addition, with the exception of grooming between a dyad that could last for several minutes, social behaviors were usually short, perhaps only a few seconds long.

However, Struhsaker carried on valiantly with his research, identifying a few more individuals as the study progressed, and following trails marked with distances so that he would know the location of the territory of each of his three main groups. He found these territorial groups to be stable from year to year, with the same adult males and females. He noted that clearly some animals preferred to be near others, but his examples comprised youngsters being close to their mothers and males hanging around a female in estrus, hoping to mate with her, rather than adults who were friends for no obvious reason. The females groomed more than did the males, while the males sometimes groomed each other but also fought; young males were driven from their group as they reached adolescence. Struhsaker saw a few embraces, such as the male CW sitting down beside the female BT, his stomach touching her right side, and putting his arms around her shoulders. Obviously, the colobus monkeys sometimes interacted in amiable dyads, but there is no way of knowing if such affectionate gestures represented a long-term special friendship, given the difficulty of carrying out observations.

PATAS MONKEYS

Naofumi Nakagawa (1992) set out to determine if there were special bonds of friendship among a group of wild patas monkeys (*Erythrocebus patas*) in the Kala Maloue National Park in northern Cameroon, during a period when the animals were not mating and not giving birth. The group comprised one adult male, three adult females, and four subadults, who lived in a prairie area where their behaviors could be observed and documented without disturbing them. He defined the four behaviors thought to portray friendship as: (a) the proximity of two animals being within three meters, (b) allogrooming that took place between dyads, (c) contact calling between two animals, and (d) animals that rested together during the night. He followed every adult all day long for two days, noting all his or her interactions with others at ten-minute intervals, as well as collecting a variety of other information.

The most striking result from the data was that the male had no preference for any of the females, for any of the four measures of interaction. He obviously liked to keep to himself.

The females were not especially friendly either. For each of the three adult female dyads, Ft and Kr, Kr and Tt, and Tt and Ft, there was no evidence of preference for any two being especially close together during their daytime activities. Any preference (greater association than would be expected above the mean) evident for any dyad included was, at most, for only two of the four parameters. Ft and Kr exchanged contact calls frequently and sometimes groomed each other preferentially; Kr and Tt sometimes groomed each other and sometimes spent the night together; and Tt and Ft sometimes called to each other, but that was all. These patas monkeys were just not much into relationships.

HAMADRYAS BABOONS

The hamadryas baboon (*Papio cynocephalus hamadryas*) was famous long before the rise of Western civilization. During Akhenaten's dynasty in Egypt, about 1350 BC, this baboon was considered sacred, an incarnation of Thoth, the god of scribes and scholars (Kummer, 1995). This belief arose, perhaps, because when males newly brought from the south were presented with writing implements, some apparently picked them up and began to scribble with them. In Egyptian tablets, a baboon is depicted sitting next to the king of the gods so that he can weigh the souls of the dead. Others, always male, are depicted as an inspirer of wisdom and a mediator between people and a god.

Up to AD 2000, it seemed unlikely that these baboons would form close friendships of any type. A mature male who remains in his natal area acquires a female when she is very young, and guards her carefully for the rest of her life, giving her neck bites if she crosses him. She is there initially by coercion (and who can tell if she would stay, given a chance to escape?). The females he gathers into his family are not related and have not grown up together, so why would they be close when they are rivals for the male's attention? As for males, they are, in large part, rivals intent on keeping their females away from other males. Hans Kummer (1968, 1995) and Jean-Jacques Abegglen (1985) both spent years studying the same baboon troops in Ethiopia, which are made up of one-male units comprising a leader male, one or more females and their young, and possibly a second or third younger follower male (who hopes eventually to take over the family himself). The relationships between these animals were visualized as a star-shaped sociogram, with the females much closer to the male leader than to each other (Kummer, 1995).

Kummer (1995) did note several examples that might be construed as amiability among males: in the Red Clan, Rosso and Rossini had such a relaxed relationship that one of them gradually relinquished his female, Rosa, to the other, and later Bub allowed one of his females, who had formerly belonged to old Rossini, to groom her erstwhile friend. A troop has no specified leader, so the males must work together to coordinate band movements during foraging, communicate directions the band should go, organize resting and watering stops, and keep individual units from becoming too dispersed (Dunbar, 1983). But the males were rivals at heart, keeping each other away from their females; males did not show altruism toward their kin, nor share meat after a hunt.

Early researchers did not focus their studies specifically on social interactions among the females, because each was thoroughly under the thumb of her male. Larissa Swedell (2002) decided to see if the females were, in fact, as little interested in each other as had been surmised. She studied hamadryas baboons living in Awash National Park, in another part of Ethiopia. Between 1996 and 1998, she spent 262 days with the baboons, following one-male units that she had habituated to her presence and recording all the activity she saw. In addition, she noted at ten-minute intervals which females were near which other individuals and which dyads were involved in grooming. In all, she collected data about 39 females from 17 one-male units (averaging 2.6 females per unit).

Swedell found that, in small units, there was little female interaction, whereas in units with more females (the maximum was five), it was greater. The females were as likely to spend time with other females as time with the male. Occasionally, a female even broke away from her unit to socialize with a female in another unit, most likely a relative with whom she was familiar. However, Swedell did not mention any two females preferring to be together rather than with other females.

In summary, both male and female hamadryas baboons got along better with members of their own sex than was originally thought, but that does not mean much. Females might have spent more time together if it were not for the jealous behavior of males, but apparently do not form fast friendships; adult males together organized the functioning of their troop, but they spent most of their time with their families. Harmony among each family unit was undermined because the females were kept under tight restraint by the much larger domineering male.

SIFAKAS

For most of the year, these arboreal lemurs (*Propithecus verreauxi verreauxi*) are placid animals who live in small groups but have little direct contact with each other. Female pairs were particularly unsocial and males, during the breeding season, actively fought with each other. Alison Jolly (1966), who watched them in Madagascar for over 250 hours in the non-breeding season, calculated that individuals interacted with each other only 0.8 times an hour. They rarely groomed each other, although they did sometimes play and wrestle in a measured way. Sifakas do, however, form what is called descriptively a "locomotive," with members of a group lining up along a strong tree branch, one animal sitting behind another with its belly pressed against the back of the one ahead and its large jumping legs enclosing him or her on either side, so that there is as much body contact as possible. The animals may sleep in this position or adopt it on a cold winter morning; however, they may also form a locomotive at noon or in hot weather.

Large herbivores

Many herbivores are classic examples of animals eating food that is readily available and not having close friendships within their groups correlated with this. This section considers giraffe, pronghorn antelope, mountain sheep, mountain goats, red deer, caribou/reindeer, white-tailed deer, African buffalo, American bison, and hippopotami.

GIRAFFE

When I studied giraffe (*Giraffa camelopardalis*) in the eastern Transvaal of South Africa in the 1950s (Innis, 1958), I should have photographed each of the 90 animals on the ranch so that I could recognize him or her individually. However, I did not have the money to buy much film nor easy access to have it processed. I did recognize some individuals by their distinctive spotting, but only a few. So I could not determine whether some pairs of animals were especially friendly with each other in that they hung around together for days and months, feeding on the leaves of trees and bushes, or resting close beside each other.

My university classmate did have these facilities in the 1960s, however. Bristol Foster made a three-year study of which individuals were present during his tour each week by vehicle through the Nairobi National Park. He accomplished this by photographing each new giraffe he saw from the left side, after searching through his earlier collection of photos to ensure that this was not an animal he already knew; the spotting on each giraffe's coat is distinctive, remaining the same throughout the animal's life. Foster could sometimes even age an individual from photos taken years earlier – when he saw a photographic postcard in a Nairobi store of the giraffe Annaliese, then young, peering at him beside an adult giraffe, he could estimate she

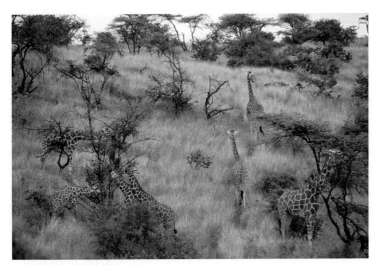

Figure 9. Giraffe do not form cohesive social groups
© photolibrary.com

was then about three years old; when he found out when the photo was taken, he knew that she was currently aged ten years (Foster, 1987).

Eventually Foster had a file of 241 individuals who had been seen in the park, some fairly often and some rarely. When we analyzed his data, recording which giraffe were present in successive weeks, we found that individual animals did not hang around together to any extent from week to week, but rather kept to their own agenda, wandering widely in the search for food or, in the case of males, for sex (Foster and Dagg, 1972).[1]

In a two-year study by Julian Fennessy (2004), of giraffe living in the Namib Desert in Namibia, southwest Africa, the density of giraffe was low given the sparse vegetation, and the herd size small – about 60 percent of giraffe sighted were in groups of three or fewer individuals. The small group sizes could reflect the limited vegetation or the lack of predation – no giraffe had been killed by lions in the previous ten years before Fennessy's research began. Solitary giraffe (usually males) were encountered most often. Some dyads of giraffe (mother and young, two subadults, or an adult and a subadult) were often seen, and in some populations, dyads of two adults also remained together for some time, but these were not numerous. Fennessy is now the Executive Director of the Kenya Land Conservation Trust, working tirelessly to prevent the nine or so subspecies or species (the taxonomic relationships are not yet clear) of giraffe from becoming extinct in Africa because of habitat reduction and increasing human populations.

PRONGHORN ANTELOPE

Female pronghorn antelope (*Antilocapra americana*) in groups look like other groups of herbivores, individuals cropping grass near each other, walking to new vegetation, feeding some more, resting together, chewing cud. What could be more idyllic? Pretty well the daily behavior of any other herbivore, John Byers (2003) discovered, as he describes in his book *Built for Speed: A Year in the Life of Pronghorn*. He spent twenty years, whenever he was not teaching at the University of Idaho, watching how pronghorn antelope behave in the National Bison Range in Montana. When interactions among individuals came thick and fast, Byers sat on the roof of his vehicle with high powered binoculars, relating who was doing what to whom while a graduate student below made frenzied notes from his descriptions.

Even though they spend almost all their time together, female pronghorn behave badly toward each other. They have a strict dominance hierarchy that persists through each animal's life. It is not based on any sort of merit, but the date when a fawn was born. A female produces two fawns in the spring, each weighing about 3.6 kg (8 lb). Each fawn begins nursing immediately, gaining about 0.23 kg (0.5 lb) a day. His or her dominance depends on weight, and thus their ability to push a smaller, younger fawn around. If you are heavier than a fawn born a day later, you can boss that youngster around every day of your life.

Picture a "herd" of female pronghorns in late summer, tired from grazing, settling down in the sun to rest at midday. A low-ranking female, such as GY, drops onto the ground near a bush. A female dominant to her, seeing this, walks threateningly toward her, forcing her to get up and move away. This female, perhaps WNB, then lies down while GY hunts for another site. Meanwhile, the more dominant DUH has noticed WNB lying down and demands that she also give up her place. Now DUH is comfortable, but GY and WNB are still looking about for a suitable grassy patch for themselves. This type of action and reaction occurs again and again in the group until all the females are at last recumbent, with the dominant ones in the center of the group. It is this configuration that the dominant animals require.

Byers, who wondered why they persisted, each day, in this anti-social behavior, decided that it evolved in prehistoric times. At present, pronghorn are so swift, sailing along at cruising speeds of up to 70 km/hr (43 mph), that no predator can hope to catch them. Ten thousand years ago, however, ancestors of pronghorn on the grass-lands of America had many predators including forebears of cheetahs, lions, and hyenas. It made sense then for individual pronghorn to stick together so that their many eyes would be likely to detect approaching danger. By forcing subordinate animals to the outside of the group at rest periods, the dominant animals made it more likely that if a lion or cheetah should attack, it would be inferior individuals rather than themselves who would serve as dinner. Obviously, female pronghorns are not into making friends with each other, given their mindset.

MOUNTAIN SHEEP

Although mountain sheep seem to lead a peaceful life, following each other about as they feed, rest, or drink, in what seems like a comradely fashion, they are actually aggressive rather than friendly. In his book *Mountain Sheep: A Study in Behavior and Evolution* (1971),

Valerius Geist describes interactions among Stone's sheep (*Ovis dalli stonei*) and among bighorn sheep (*Ovis canadensis canadensis*). To begin his years of research that would earn him his doctorate in zoology, he built himself a small hut near the timber line in northern British Columbia in which to live. There the temperature was incredibly cold during the winter, but if a sudden chinook storm blew in from the Pacific, it could raise the temperature from −40°F to +40°F in a few hours. Each day he observed and noted down sheep activity. The Stone's sheep in the pristine wilderness, all extremely wary of people because of hunting pressure, had varied coat colors and horn sizes and shapes, which enabled him to recognize a number of individuals. In Banff National Park further south where no hunting was allowed, the bighorn sheep were so accustomed to humans that, far from fleeing at Geist's approach on foot, they hurried toward him to lick the salt blocks that he placed on the ground. While individuals licked the salt, he read the small marking tags within their ears. He could age rams (but not ewes) roughly from the size of their horns.

Groups of males and of females with their young kept largely to themselves during most of the year, coming together only in the fall for the mating season, so there are no long-term male–female pairs. This separation of the sexes after the rut ensures that the males do not consume resources needed by the females and their developing fetuses (Geist and Petocz, 1977). For both species, Geist (1971) noted whenever he saw one of 13 behaviors between two sheep, male or female, most of which were antagonistic (such as front kick, butt, horn thrust, clash), some sexual (mounting, sniffing rear, Flehmen), and only two somewhat friendly (horning the body and rubbing). By far the most common non-sexual behaviors of males of both species toward females were a low-stretch horn display, a twist–threat display, or a front kick. None would encourage friendly feelings. The dominant males never rubbed against the females or lightly horned their bodies, as females did to them when they were in estrus. When females were not in estrus, they kept out of the way of the rams.

How did males, who spent most of the year together, act toward one another? They had a dominance hierarchy based, in large part, on size, with the larger or dominant animals treating the smaller or subordinate ones in the same negative way they treated females, including mounting them (in homosexual behavior). By contrast, the smaller rams seemed desperate to befriend the larger ones. Their three most common contact behaviors were nuzzling, horning, and rubbing their target. Nuzzling involved approaching the larger ram to lick and nuzzle his head; horning was touching his horn to the face, chest, or shoulder of his elder; and rubbing involved rubbing his face on the face of the dominant animal, perhaps picking up scent from his scent glands. Thus, for both Stone's and bighorn sheep, the dominant rams were likely to threaten the subordinate ones, while the subordinate rams tried to curry favor with their betters or at least get their attention, as they also sometimes butted or clashed against the dominant's well-armored head. Rams became even less social as they aged and were more often seen alone.

Among females, relations were also sour. For both Stone's and bighorn sheep, the most common interactions were low-stretch horn displays, butts, rushes, and horn threats. The somewhat friendly behaviors of rubbing and horning were almost non-existent. At least the females did not become more lonely as they aged. The evidence indicates that female bighorn and Stone's sheep, like the males, do not really like each other. Sheep tolerate each other because they feed in the same areas. They are gregarious because it is safer to be so when there is danger from predators such as wolves, cougars, and bears.

How did such gregariousness evolve? Geist postulates that it was a two-fold response to the environment and to early training of the young. Mountain sheep graze on a home range comprising stable grasslands and alpine vegetation present within mountain ranges. Young animals who are gregarious by nature stay within the foraging area along with their elders, while the more adventuresome young who disperse are unlikely to thrive. The same home range is thus passed from one generation to the next. After weaning in the fall, the bond between mother and young becomes tenuous. This means that the mothers do not need to drive their yearlings away when their next offspring is born, thus forcing them from the home range. A youngster may no longer follow its mother, but rather trail along after other sheep to another group. Early behavior has offspring following their mothers to be close to their source of milk, and the ewes staying near the lambs to reduce the pressure of milk in their udders. When the mother is in estrus, she searches out large males to follow, and a line of often smaller males follows her, attracted by her condition. Youth follows age, but even aging ewes follow other sheep. Most sheep stay together, but that does not mean they have to like each other.

In his more recent 10-year research on bighorn sheep in southwest Alberta, Marco Festa-Bianchet (1991) also found that female relatives did not support or become friendly with each other as they do in many species, and he suggests four reasons why amicable behavior did not evolve:

(a)   vegetation for the sheep is spread out so that it cannot be defended to benefit a relative;

(b)   ewes do not defend cooperatively against coyote attack, but rather flee with their lambs;

(c)   relatives do not help each other with aggressive interactions against other sheep; and

(d)   there is little opportunity for coalitions of related females to help each other to increase their reproductive performance; dominance, for example, had no apparent effect on reproductive success. Bighorn sheep are gregarious because of predation, despite the disadvantages of competition for forage and parasitic transmission, but there was no special benefit in being gregarious with relatives rather than with non-relatives. More than five sheep are needed in a group to be above the threshold where alertness against predators can decline for each animal and feeding rate increase, but there were not five relatives in a group to effect this advantage.

MOUNTAIN GOATS

Sociality (but not gregariousness) among female mountain goats (*Oreamnos americanus*) is as negative as that among pronghorns or bighorn sheep. Marco Festa-Bianchet and Steeve Côté (2008), in their book *Mountain Goats: Ecology, Behavior, and Conservation of an Alpine Ungulate*, describe the research they have carried out, over 15 years, on the social behavior and other aspects of an unhunted population in the foothills of the Rocky Mountains of west-central Alberta. Their initial aim was to capture and mark every animal in the population so that they could recognize it from a distance. They did this by using blocks of salt in huts set up as traps, or under drop nets where the goats came to lick the salt. The goats were fitted with numbered or colored tags in their ears, regular collars, or collars with radio transmitters so that the location of the animal could be traced. In all, 210 mountain goats were given functioning radio collars over the years, but the use of such manipulations sometimes skewed the research results.[2]

The researchers obtained little information on sociality among males, because outside of the rutting period, the billies hung out alone or with only a few other males, the size of the groups decreasing leading up to the fall rut when the males joined the females for the mating season. In addition, they tended to stay in forested areas – some marked individuals were only seen four or five times or not at all during a season.

Because of these problems, the researchers focused their efforts on the females who were more gregarious and more visible. Groups of nannies and their young were small at first, but increased in size during the summer. The nannies (like the males in their groups) had a linear dominance hierarchy, which meant that when two individuals of the same sex came near each other, the subordinate one virtually always gave way without question; all adult goats are aggressive, with sharp horns that can deliver serious or fatal stab wounds should there be a physical confrontation, so the most dominant animals tend to be the oldest. Rarely, one nanny might rush at and menace another with her horns, but usually such open threats were unnecessary because each individual knew her place.

Given their truculence, perhaps it is not surprising that the mountain goats did not have preferred adult partners with whom they spent time, not even if relatives, such as mothers and daughters, were in a group. Why should this be so, as kin in many species often provide support to each other, to their mutual genetic benefit? There may be several reasons. Because of the extreme climate and terrain of this species, reproduction rate is low compared to other ungulates, with infant mortality fairly high, so there are few close relatives in any one group. Because the larger a group's size, the more effective it is against predators, these few relatives probably would not be able to help each other to avoid predation, particularly against cougars which attack by ambush. Indeed, mountain goats have no group defence of any sort against predators except flight. In addition, food and water are spread out, so again there would be no possibility of one animal helping another to access these resources.

Far from leading a peaceful existence in majestic mountains, snacking together on tasty vegetation, and resting with each other in a companionable way, the females spent far more time than most social ungulates in harassing or being harassed by their neighbors (Fournier and Festa-Bianchet, 1995). The rates of aggressive interactions between mountain goat female pairs were more than three times those for female pairs of roe deer and feral horses, and over five times those for female pairs of red deer, bison, chamois, and bighorn sheep.

RED DEER

European red deer (*Cervus elaphus*), the same species as the North American elk, are relatively easy to research – they are large, have a fairly short lifespan, live in open habitats, and if not hunted, are fairly easily habituated to human observers. They were one of the first mammals to have their activities studied in detail. Fraser Darling, with a background in agriculture and an interest in animal behavior, was thrilled to be encouraged to do this in Scotland. His book *A Herd of Red Deer: A Study in Animal Behaviour* was published in 1937. He was notable for putting the boot to the romantic ideal of "Monarch of the Glen" – that a mighty stag was the leader of any red deer herd. In reality, large herds made up of hinds and their young are always led by a mature or old female who has a youngster at heel. The egocentric stags form much looser herds with no leader at all, but often a few bullies. They tolerate each other for most of the year, but fight fiercely during the rutting season for the privilege of mating with females.[3]

Nearly half a century after Darling's study, Tim Clutton-Brock and his colleagues (1982) launched a second research project on red deer, lasting ten years this time and much more ambitious because of far better financing. Clutton-Brock is a British zoologist based at Cambridge University, well known for his research into the social behavior of primates and meerkats (where his favorites appeared in the television program *Meerkat Manor*), as well as red deer. The study region for his red deer research was a section of the Isle of Rhum, west Scotland, where a few hundred animals roamed. The men soon recognized all of the individuals in the area based on facial features, body shape, coat color, and antler shapes (male), along with the help of ear flashes, and expandable collars on many of the young. They carried out up to five censuses a month, recording the identity, position, activity, and location of all deer in view. In addition, some individuals were followed for a whole day and night, the observers noting what each was doing every minute or, after dark, every five minutes using infrared viewing equipment. This required four-hour shifts for from two to four observers at a time. The nearest two neighboring deer of the target animal were identified, which enabled the researchers to determine if he or she had preferred friends with whom to hang out. The "nearest neighbor distance" was defined as "the linear distance between the head of an animal and the head of the animal nearest to it excluding its own calf."

The two sexes kept to themselves throughout most of the year, roaming in parties defined as aggregations "where no individual was more than 50 meters [55 yd] from any other animal in the same party." Those often present in the same party were considered associates. The stags and hinds only joined together in the fall for the mating season, so there were no long-term male–female partnerships. Nor did it seem that females chose one stag rather than another to approach for copulation, although they did prefer older to younger mates.

The hinds tended to cluster with matriline relatives in small parties of up to seven animals, whose composition was often stable from year to year. In one table in which the authors compare dyads of relatives of animals over two years of age, during two years of observations, mothers were associated with adult daughters 139 times, sisters with sisters 58 times, aunts with nieces 47 times, and grandmothers with granddaughters 18 times. These numbers are not definitive, but give an idea of the relative importance of genetic relationships or of being raised in the same group, and thus familiar with relatives since birth. The hinds in matriline parties got along fairly well, feeding sometimes with heads only a few centimeters apart, with few threats between individuals. However, there were also few direct interactions among the hinds; rarely one hind licked or nibbled another's head and neck, but this attention was not reciprocated. There were also occasional conflicts within a herd between females related to the dominance hierarchy; older hinds were likely to win, even though younger animals might be physically larger (Thouless and Guinness, 1986). Clutton-Brock and his colleagues (1982) do not report noticing any especially close relationships between two individuals. However, herd members kept unrelated females away from their grazing grounds and orphan females were often threatened, forced to move away from feeding areas, and less likely to be made aware by herd hinds of danger from predators.

Unlike the female groups, the males in the stag groups were usually unrelated, because when they had been old enough to leave their natal range, they had gravitated to different core areas. Even grown brothers were not interested in each other, sometimes to the point of fighting. The male herds were looser than those of the females, individuals joining or leaving a group from hour to hour, with stags farther apart and threatening each other three times as often as did the females among themselves. During the rutting season, stags were obsessed with trying to keep their "harems" together and other males away from the females; this caused much chasing and fighting among the eventually exhausted dominant males. When they grew old, the stags often became loners. Like mountain sheep, red deer may look peaceable in their herds, but there is tension running through them that may erupt into threats and fights, especially among the stags.

WHITE-TAILED DEER

White-tailed deer (*Odocoileus virginianus*) do not have preferred companions with whom they interact closely year after year. After the fall breeding season in the northern part of their range in North America, deer often gather in fairly large numbers in wintering yards of cedar swamps and dense vegetation, but they do so not because they like each other's company, but because they are protected there from bitter winds and deep snow (Thomas, 2009). The rest of the year they return to the familiar terrain they regard as home. The females move in family groups with their young, but when a new fawn or fawns are born in the spring, they chase away their yearlings who must then fend for themselves. The males remain alone or hang out loosely with other males during the spring and summer, but in the autumn they become fierce rivals for the opportunity to mate with females.

AFRICAN BUFFALO

Except for very old pairs near the end of their lives (see the chapter: *Old buddies*), African buffalo may associate in herds of many hundreds of animals, so members of this species obviously have a tendency to follow each other and to associate in large aggregations. Herbert Prins of the Netherlands (1996), who watched and recorded buffalo activity in the Lake Manyara National Park in Tanzania for many years, asserts in his thoughtful book *Ecology and Behaviour of the African Buffalo* that herds are large because, at least for the females, they can share information about the best grazing grounds and reduce their danger of being killed by lions.

How does this sharing information work? After two years of observation, Prins finally figured out what was happening. "Voting" about where to graze that evening took place in the afternoon, when the 950 Manyara buffalo were lying down and resting, usually on the mudflats along the lake shore. Shortly after five o'clock, a few cows became restive, stood up facing a certain direction with their heads lifted rather high, and then bedded down again after a minute or so. Until six o'clock, a few cows did this sequentially, most roughly gazing toward the same place. At this time, as the shadow of the escarpment to the west moved over the herd as the sun went down, the animals began to rouse themselves. In a few minutes they were all standing, and shortly after this they began to trek in the direction indicated, as if by consensus obtained from the voting animals. No particular individual led; on average, the individual at the head of a group changed every minute for cows, and every fifteen minutes for bulls; subadult animals were never in the lead.

As the buffalo traveled to the new feeding ground, they did so in a specific formation that usually remained fixed for a female. The males and females in the best condition walked in the front half of the herd (except at the very front where there is danger from lions), while those who were less fit brought up the rear; by virtue of their position, the rearguard ate less nutritious food and suffered from larger infestations of intestinal nematodes present in the numerous fecal pats dropped by their betters. The latter group did not defect from the herd to form a new one, because they valued the information about grazing locations shared by other females in the voting procedure: "As perfect information is hardly ever available to one individual, information sharing can lead to better decisions." Because Prins was unable to identify most of the myriad of individuals, he could not determine if some females might have preferred partners. Probably not, because a female's place in the herd formation changed with her reproductive condition (producing a calf, having her calf die, or weaning the calf), and he did not report that another female changed her position to be near a friend.

For a herd of about 100 buffalo (*Syncerus caffer caffer*) studied for several years in south-western Kenya, Mark Mloszewski (1983) did observe some interactions among females, although he was unable to recognize all of the animals individually. For example, in one subgroup the top three dominant animals (whose dominance was tested when two individuals had a spat and the subordinate one withdrew) were, in order, the high-status, elderly but energetic PE, the younger MD, and the strong PV. MD, who was younger than the other two, may have been a daughter of PE. PV won some of her encounters against PE, but lost those against MD. When PE was shot, however, MD lost her status so that PV became the alpha cow. Mloszewski hypothesizes that because of the close friendship or relationship between PE and MD, MD had "borrowed" status from the older PE. With PE gone, she lost it again, her rank was down-graded and she became subordinate to PV, and apparently some of her relatives. Further research may show that some females do have special friendships.

Among prime males, Prins found that dyads were rarely seen together for more than a day, or only a few hours, so there were certainly no stable associations. The males often left a herd to hang around in small bachelor groups of about three, or to travel to another herd to try to find a female in estrus with whom to mate. The males, who are far larger (about 650 kg or 1430 lb) than the females (under 500 kg or 1100 lb), are often alone, and for this reason they are much more vulnerable to lion attack than are the cows in their large aggregations.

Mloszewski did notice a few male affiliations for buffalo living in Zambia. For example, four males (A, B, C, D) who had broken away from their larger group had, at first, a definite linear hierarchy from A to D. Two days later and from then on, B and D kept close company while A remained dominant to the three others, and B was dominant still to C and D. However, D started to behave in a dominant manner toward C. Mloszewski hypothesizes that D had borrowed status because of his relationship with B and was then able to boss C about. Apparently, such affiliations can affect an individual's dominance ranking.

AMERICAN BISON

Female American bison (*Bison bison*) and their young, unlike the males, live in large nomadic herds that now slowly wander and graze over the reduced grass plains of mid-west America. During the rutting season, the males join with these herds in hopes of mating with a cow in estrus, although there is not a lot of mating going on; most females accept only one male partner, perhaps because his quick, final pelvic thrust ends with his whole one-ton (900 kg) weight on her hindquarters (Lott, 2002). With so little sex available, all the adult males become fierce rivals during the rut, their aggression exacerbated by females in estrus who run through a herd as if to announce their receptive condition and foment competition, in which they fully succeed.

Outside the rutting season, males are more pacific, but not very friendly. Dale Lott (2002), in his book *American Bison*, describes two old bulls lying down near each other before the rutting season, resting and chewing their cud. One stands, stretches, and looks around; then the other does, too. When the first male approaches the second, a slight tension develops between them; they stare at each other, then slowly relax. They amble about one hundred meters (110 yd) while grazing, then lie down again. The following day, one may have joined several other bulls, and the other may be alone, but they will both still be eating, ruminating, and resting, putting on weight that will help them through the rut and the long winter season to follow.

What about friendship between cows? Lott states that the bond between a mother and her calf, which lasts for the six months leading up to weaning, is by far the strongest and longest in a buffalo's life. This indicates that bonds between two cows are slight or non-existent. It would be difficult even to discover such friendships, given that the bison lifestyle involves the cows slowly walking and grazing, along with their calves, close together but not too close, for hundreds of miles each year. There is a dominance relationship between individual bison as well, which can work against special friendships. Where food is abundant, such as on the National Bison Range in Montana, dominance relationships are more or less in abeyance, so that little aggression is in evidence. Where food is limited, as on Catalina Island, California, however, dominance means superiority and is correlated with weight – the larger the cow, the more she can get what she wants, eating the best food and drinking first at water sites – figuratively throwing her weight around.

CARIBOU AND REINDEER

It would be impossible to follow caribou (*Rangifer tarandus*) day after day to determine if there are, among the enormous number of animals who make up their herds, preferred partners – individuals who like to walk together side by side or feed nose-to-nose. We should not think of caribou as migrating from one area to another, a wildlife professor once announced to my class at university, but of them stopping their incessant travel now and then for such things as browsing or giving birth. What caribou do all year long is move forward – in part because all the members of their huge herds would not be able to find enough food in any one place. So caribou are very gregarious, but do they have special friends?

Researchers *have* been able to study the social behavior of reindeer in Finland, where the animals belong to the same species but are semi-domesticated. If reindeer are not very social, then likely caribou who live in the North American arctic are not either. This makes sense, because it is surely especially difficult to instigate and maintain a friendship while on the hoof, day after day, for a lifetime.

Akira Hirotani (1990) carried out nine months of observation on reindeer groups living in five enclosures within a 46 square kilometer (18 sq mi) area in Finnish Lapland. Along with many fawns, there were about 110 females one year of age or older, each recognized individually because of body size, body color, shape of antlers, ear tags, or plastic collars; there were also ten males aged two years or older, and several castrated males. The females arranged themselves into a dominance hierarchy based largely on size, which Hirotani could decipher by noting who won the many antagonistic interactions that included charging, chasing, sparring, and displacement of others at resting places or feeding craters. Hirotani also recorded, for all the dyads in the five herds, how often these two individuals were seen together using an Association Index.

The results indicated that unrelated females did not hang out with preferred partners in the various groups that formed and reformed from time to time. Nor did mothers show preference for their daughters as they grew to adulthood. They were particularly antagonistic against their yearling daughters when their next fawn was born; the more a yearling sought to be with her mother, the more her mother attacked her, whereas mothers without new fawns remained friendly with their year-old daughters. Reindeer, like caribou, live in a harsh, unforgiving environment. During winter, both eat lichens under the snow by digging craters at which the fawns feed along with their mothers; if the reindeer mothers had maintained their close bond with their yearling daughters once they had new fawns, this might have put the infants in jeopardy because of feeding-crater competition.

Nor were females friendly toward males. Males were dominant to females during the rut while they both had antlers, but the males lost theirs soon after while the females did not. The females then became largely dominant during the winter, winning about 80 percent of antagonistic interactions, with even young females attacking adult males. Caribou, like reindeer, are gregarious, but it is almost certain that they also lack stable social relationships within their herds.

Hippopotami

How do you study the behavior of hippopotami? Researcher Stewart Eltringham (1999) says, with difficulty. If you lob paint at an individual it soon wears off, and anyway cannot be seen well in murky water or at night when the animals come onto the shore to graze. If you try to tranquilize them with a dart, it may not go through the thick skin, or it may paralyze only part of the animal (in one case the hind quarters which left the huge mouth anxious to bite anyone who came close). If the drug does start to take effect, the hippopotamus may rush into the water and drown, or if it is on land, it can be difficult to follow in the dark. Ear tags fall off as hippopotami shake their heads, collars slip over their heads because their large necks are so slippery, and radio transmitters do not function well when immersed in water. Researchers therefore must go with size and what distinctive natural markings are recognizable. Despite these difficulties, Eltringham was able to identify many individual hippopotami and document their activities in and near lakes and along stretches of rivers in Africa.

Like elephants and orcas, hippopotami (*Hippopotamus amphibius*) also live in tight aggregations, although unlike these behemoths, they do not move about from place to place seeking food but, aside from dispersals by the young, stay in the same small area during their entire adult lifespan (Eltringham, 1999; Feldhake, 2005). If they are sleeping on the shore during the heat of the day, their bodies are close enough to be touching. When they are in water, which is most of the time, they are always in a crowd. Yet at heart they are asocial animals. Alpha males are psychically solitary individuals albeit surrounded by other hippopotami; they fiercely fight any male challenger who tries to take over their territory, although they do not worry about young males who are neither rivals nor friendly with each other. Females are not interested in the males and may return after a night of grazing to another territory entirely, with a different alpha male. Females also show little concern for each other, although they may nurse calves who are not their own; field studies report that the number of lactating females may be two or three times the number of young nursing calves in the population (Feldhake, 2005). At night when females go onto land to feed, they may leave their calves in the care of other females. However, Eltringham states categorically that there are no social bonds between adults.

MEERKATS

Until recently, little was known about the social behavior of small mammals in the wild because they were too difficult to observe. This changed when Tim Clutton-Brock decided to do a long-term study on diminutive meerkats (*Suricata suricatta*), which live in family groups in open areas of southern Africa. They became habituated to human beings to such an extent as to be trained to step onto scales for a sip of water or a bit of egg, to be weighed both before and after foraging to determine how much they ate. Over 14 years, Clutton-Brock and over 50 volunteers came to know 300 meerkats individually, living in 14 groups. He has described his findings in a TV program and in a wonderful book entitled *Meerkat Manor: Flower of the Kalahari* (2007), Flower being a dominant female who led her family group for most of her life, before she died of snake-bite at the age of seven years. All of the 37 members of her group at the time, except for the dominant male, were either her children or her grandchildren.

Meerkats always live in a group because they need many members to feed their infants and to watch constantly for predators while foraging. Even so, and perhaps because of these imperatives, their social system is such that members never become close friends. Instead, social concourse is a mixture of extreme cooperation between individuals, probably greater than that in any other species, and ruthless conflict. Take the females who are usually related as sisters, mothers, and daughters. They are seemingly congenial at times, some baby-sitting and even nursing the newborns when their mothers and the others are out foraging; they willingly donate insects and scorpions to youngsters old enough to straggle after the group when the adults are feeding.

However, at other times the females are at each other's throats. Dominant females such as Flower thought nothing of shoving aside a comrade to steal a tasty millipede she or he was digging up. When her group became too large, she attacked and drove out adult females, including her own progeny, to fend for themselves. Flower tried desperately to prevent even her daughters from breeding so that her own young could survive. During the reproductive season, females become competitors, "chattering at each other and hip-slamming their rivals as they walked past." If four or five females become pregnant at about the same time, some of these will kill the young of the first female to give birth. The same thing happens to the infants of the second female. Only the last female to give birth produces young who are allowed to live.

Nor do other types of dyads get along. Males fight fiercely among themselves to increase their rank in the dominance hierarchy; they are opportunistic in their challenges, often waiting until a rival is ill or exhausted after a fight before attacking. Because their daughters do not mate with them when they reach maturity, males disperse from their group to find other females in estrus with whom to mate. A male and a female are equally unsociable; females will mate with a number of males, but they do not spend time with them.

This chapter about social animals who are uncongenial seems an oddity in a book devoted to special friendships, but the content is of interest because it sheds light on why close bonds do not take place, and therefore what features *do* foster bonds between individuals. The following chapter considers friendships between animals of two different species. These alliances are almost unknown for adults in the wild, but do occur sometimes between an adult and an infant (which are not relevant here), and between wild and domestic adults. When they do occur, such friendships shed light on the psyches of the participants.

Cross-species pals

Hundreds of social species mingle freely with other social species if they are not predators (which, by contrast, except for lions are usually solitary rather than gregarious). Zebras forage alongside wildebeest, waterfowl and shore birds of many species mix together, colonial species of marine birds crowd on cliff faces, and a variety of birds gather at bird feeding stations. Such sociality may stress feeding resources, but it improves safety for the many animals. Here, however, we are interested in special friendships between two or a few adults of different species.

Newspapers often run fetching pictures of two such adult animals cozying up together (and many more involving a cute infant, which do not concern us here). In my "Interspecies Friends" file I have best buddy photographs of a Siamese cat and a parrot, a red setter and a hamster, two swans and a goose, a deer and a horse, a poodle and a budgie, dogs and rabbits, a dog and a fawn, and a cat and a squirrel, all taken by or for the proud human companions of these odd couples. Often one of these animals was an orphaned youngster when it met its pal; if animals become familiar with each other from an early age, they are often fast friends for life. Early experiments have shown that when a kitten is raised with a rat, the cat will not kill its friend, even though it may kill other rats (Kuo, 1930). Animal Sanctuaries are where such curious friendships flourish, genial homes as they are to needy animals of various species (Hatkoff, 2009).

Other photographs and news stories in my file are of a domestic or farm animal along with a wild one:

- A domestic cow and moose bull became famous, in 1986, for hanging out together on a Vermont farm, the status of their close friendship reported every few weeks in the news. On the 77th day of their first encounter, the moose dropped his antlers, and the next morning walked away from his Jessica. Wildlife biologists suggested that the two and a half-year-old male may have been attracted to Jessica when she was in estrus, and remained as her buddy when she was no longer in heat. When he lost his antlers, though, he also lost his sex drive and his intense attraction to the cow. A song "Lovesick Moose" commemorates their friendship.

- A young, originally orphaned baboon in Namibia accompanied a flock of goats, which went out to pasture each day with her riding on the back of one of the billies (who are larger and more stable than the nannies), sitting up when they ambled along and lying down if they ran. She was fed at night, but also picked up tidbits of vegetation from her high perch or the ground during the day. The farmers in the area told researchers S. P. Henzi and A. MacDonald (1986), perhaps tongue-in-cheek, that baboons often acted as shepherds to flocks of goats, ideal in that they were careful custodians who never took time off, received no pay, and never had hangovers.

- A cat and a groundhog kept company for an entire summer on the property of the novelist Timothy Findley (1998). During a dry spell, the groundhog first followed Moth to his house. After she had taken a drink from her water bowl on the porch while the

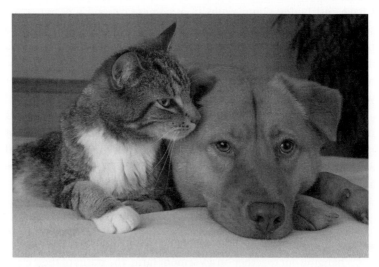

Figure 10. Even two predators can be best friends.
© istockphoto.com/Michael Pettigrew

groundhog sat back on its haunches watching, it drank there too. The groundhog continued to live in the pasture on the other side of the road, but it visited its friend many times during the summer; perhaps looking for a drink of water as well?

Other unusual groupings include:

- Three amigos: Each winter near Vancouver for seven years, especially during the annual Christmas bird count, birders were thrilled once again to see the three amigos, three large shore birds that hung out together there – a long-billed curlew, a whimbrel, and a marbled godwit, each a rarity in its own right. There used to be a willet, too, making up the Gang of Four, but it disappeared (Whelan, 1997).
- Robins and cardinals: One nest near Cincinnati was shared by three northern cardinal and four robin nestlings. All four parents worked together to bring food for the youngsters, but each species was inclined to give precedence to its own brood (Broadminded robins, 2002).
- Chimpanzee and olive baboon: While settling down by a large *Cordia* tree in the Kibale Forest of Uganda to watch chimpanzees come to feed, Michael Ghiglieri (1988) was amazed to see a baboon hanging out with the high-ranking male chimpanzee, Silverback. He had not seen Silverback for months. The odd couple climbed into the tree, moved to opposite sides of it following chimpanzee protocol, and began eating the date-like fruit. Baboons were numerous in the forest, perhaps because they were more vulnerable on savanna lands to men who hunted them, but they were almost impossible to observe. When the baboon spotted Ghiglieri, he fled, barking a warning to Silverback who paid no attention. Ghiglieri suspected that the baboon had left his last troop and was hunting for a new one to join.

It is no surprise that two animals brought into close contact can, in effect, sometimes "fall in love with each other." This happens all the time between people and their companion animals, even though the person may not use these words. In his book *The Pig Who Sang to the Moon* about the emotional lives of farm animals, Jeffrey Masson (2003) mentions a number of cross-species' bonds: a Muscovy duck with a chicken, a chicken with a turkey, pigs individually with dogs (pigs are very social and friendly by nature), and a turkey and people. Many race horses like to have special friends near them at their home barn and in their racing box: a sheep, a goat, a donkey, and even a rabbit (although there were problems when the rabbit gave birth to a large litter) (Dower, 1998). One horse, Murphy, was happy to have a wild turkey stand on his back (Linden, 1999). When the turkey wandered up, Murphy lowered his head so that his friend could climb aboard. This strange friendship lasted for about a year.

Sometimes pair-associations are solid but lopsided. Masson (2003) met a cow, Whisper, who had been born blind in rural Missouri. She was friends with a two-year-old ram, Rammo, who acted as her protector. He fed beside her in the pasture each day, making sure she did not bump into posts or fences. When someone called Whisper's name, she looked around expectantly; she did not seem to realize that she was different than the other animals around her. When she gave birth to a calf, Shout, Rammo looked out for him too, although he had no time for the lambs he himself sired.

A similar relationship existed between the blind mule Annie and her sighted and constant companion Charlie, a steer, both residents of Colorado's Black Forest Animal Sanctuary (Bekoff, 2007). They were kept in separate paddocks, so did not meet until one winter which was so cold that all the animals were herded into a single pen to keep warm. Charlie was immediately taken with Annie. He nuzzled up to her, played with her, and stayed near her. From then on, he led her each day to the water tank and around the pasture so she could avoid the fences. They also slept close beside each other.

COYOTES AND BADGERS

Coyotes and badgers (*Taxidea taxus*) are mortal enemies and rivals: coyotes kill badgers, especially young ones; both are predators of small mammals; but they can also be buddies. In Wyoming, Steve Minta implanted radio transmitters under the skin of badgers (they do not have a long enough neck to be able to wear a collar) so that he could find out more about their lives (Lott, 2002). Often their radio signals led him to a colony of ground squirrels where there was a coyote hanging about. Many times Minta sat back and watched what was happening through his binoculars. The badger was digging into the homes of the ground squirrels and eating any that he came across. The ground squirrels that fled were captured by the coyote, who ate them as well. It was a win-win situation for the predators (but hell for the squirrels) – the rodents were more reluctant to escape into the jaws of the coyote than to stay in their tunnels, so the badger had a good meal, while any that did rush out gave the coyote more food than he would have had without the badger's help.

This scenario was more than mere symbiosis. The usually solitary badger and the coyote had a relationship. The coyote always initiated their joint adventure with his usual repertoire of behaviors: play-bowing to the badger, wagging his tail, and scampering about excitedly. The badger responded, even though adult badgers do not invite other badgers to play. They both bounced about for a bit before touching noses, somehow indicating that they were no longer enemies, but partners in a shared gastronomic adventure. Then the badger began his digging. When they took a break from the hunt, the two animals rested to digest their meals, sometimes their bodies touching as they snoozed on the ground.

AN ELEPHANT AND A DOG

At an elephant retirement sanctuary in Tennessee, each new arrival searches for a special friend to chum with (CBS News, 2009.01.02). The 3950 kg (8700 lb) Tarra found Bella, one of the dozen stray dogs that hung out there. Co-founder of the sanctuary Carol Buckley notes that Tarra knows she is not a dog, and Bella knows she is not an elephant, but they have still got along fine for years, eating, drinking, sleeping, and playing together. When Bella suffered a spinal cord injury, the depth of their friendship became apparent. Rather than roam in the sanctuary, Tarra spent each day near the office where Bella lay paralyzed. After a few weeks, Bella was carried to the balcony so she and Tarra could see each other. Bella began feebly to wag her tail, so she was taken down to visit with the elephant. After that they visited each day until Bella was able to walk again. The elephant and the dog remain fast friends, Tarra sometimes rubbing Bella's stomach with her enormous foot. The news item ends: "Just two living creatures who somehow managed to look past their immense differences. Take a good look at this couple, America. Take a good look world. If they can do it – what's our excuse?"

ZOO WOLF AND GOATS

By their very definition, social animals are tolerant of other animals and often keen for friendship. In zoos and barnyards, even members of unrelated species may choose to become close buddies as we have seen. In his book *The Parrot's Lament*, Eugene Linden (1999) describes a timber wolf in the San Diego Zoo who lived in a large enclosure next to that shared by two Cretan goats. Soon they became familiar with each other, then three fast friends, tearing back and forth along the fence that kept them apart, the goats jumping and bouncing as if in full flight, the wolf loping beside them. While they rested, the wolf tried to lick the faces of his friends through the fence mesh. Soon, the keeper was letting them out at the same time each day so they could frolic together. She could only persuade the wolf back into his quarters at nightfall after the goats had been safely shut away. Linden notes that by seeming to chase the goats, the wolf feels like a real wolf, even though they are his friends, and by rushing about the goats become energized but not a meal. Animals in zoos often try to express themselves as best they can under trying conditions.

CATS AND DOGS

People who have cats and dogs do not usually think about how amazing this is, that two unrelated "predators" should be able to coexist more or less peacefully in close quarters, often becoming best buddies. The dog has a history of human contact going back many thousands of years, contact which involved significant amounts of selective breeding. By contrast, the cat has been closely involved with people for a much shorter time. A dog's life is closely intertwined with that of his human companions, who are in effect his pack, while a cat is content to go his or her own way.

What about the adage "they fought like dogs and cats"? No way. To study this relationship in depth, graduate student Neta-li Feuerstein and professor Joseph Terkel (2008) carried out a two-pronged study in Tel Aviv. The first was having a questionnaire filled in by 170 people who had both cats and dogs living with them, asking about the behavior of these animals toward each other. The second was direct observation of dog and cat interactions in 45 households by the two researchers and a householder. (Who ever said that science was boring?) The householder guided the researchers to a closed room with a cat and a dog present ten minutes before observations were begun, so that the animals could sniff, lick, and rub against each other to become reacquainted. Five minutes into the observation period, the householder rolled a tennis ball between the animals to see if they would play together, or if one animal would dominate any interaction. Then the householder played with them to elicit other behaviors, all of which were categorized as either amicable, aggressive, or indifferent.

During these experiments, the researchers video-taped (with two cameras) everything that occurred. They were keen to know if each animal had learned the body language of the other from living together (Science News, 2008). For example, cats tend to lash their tails when they are angry, while dogs arch their backs. When it is happy, a cat purrs while a dog wags its tail. A cat indicates aggression when it averts its head, while a dog signals submission with the same posture.

The researchers found that most dogs and cats got along fine, often playing and sleeping together. Sometimes they groomed each other and shared the same water dish. They often sniffed nose-to-nose, an example of a social interaction that does not exist in a dog's natural repertoire and, therefore, had had to be acquired by the dog. Male and female dogs were equally friendly with a cat of either sex, but female cats tended to be more aggressive or indifferent to dogs than did tom cats. This was surprising, because in nature the female cat is less antagonistic than the male. Most of the females had been neutered, which usually makes them less aggressive to other cats, so the researchers suggest that the neutering may instead have made them more aggressive to other species, even if not to their own.

The order of adoption influenced how well the dog and cat got along. If the dog had been first, he or she showed greater aggression or indifference to a cat brought home later than if the cat had been adopted first. The dog who had been well ensconced in the family seemed to be displaying jealousy about the cat and the attention it received, just as he or she did if a new baby were brought into a home. The cat did not care whether or not a dog was present when it was adopted, behaving the same way toward it no matter what. As a solitary species, the cat has little psychic dependency on its human companions and was not upset if a dog was later added to the household.

Most dogs and cats living together amicably showed an equal ability to understand each other's body language, the dog learning "cat" language and the cat, "dog." This was especially true if they became acquainted when young, ideally up to age six months for the cat and up to one year for the dog. In the same way, they have learned to understand the behavior and commands of their human companions – Walkies? Hungry? Down boy! (Strangely, our own dog, Sport, went berserk with happiness in anticipation of a walk when he heard the word "archipelago.")

The researchers conclude their article on a practical note, observing that domestic cats like to have another animal around, judging from their then higher scores of amiable behavior. Therefore, it makes sense to adopt a dog facing euthanization from an animal shelter to keep the cat company (Science News, 2008). They also note optimistically that if members of different species of predators can learn to live together harmoniously, then surely the same should be true of humans belonging to a single species, whether neighbors, work colleagues, or statesmen.

In summary, a few animals become buddies with individuals of another species, but these associations are rare, occurring usually under unnatural conditions. They do emphasize the central importance companionship and close bonds have to many individuals.

The final chapter discusses relationships between animals and people. In her book *Made for Each Other* (2009), Meg Daley Olmert is remarkably sanguine about our non-human friendships. She writes: "We and other mammals have a common social biology that allows us to approach, interact, and relax in each other's company" and that, in the olden days, once we began to interact, "an interspecies culture based on cooperation and contentment" was created. When one recalls how people have treated animals over the years, with mass slaughters, factory farms, circus and rodeo abuses, and destruction of habitat, it is difficult to agree with her thesis. However, there have been a number of close pairings between humans and mammals or birds, some of which are described in the last chapter.

Animal and human "friendships"

"Animals are such agreeable friends – they ask no questions, they pass no criticisms," George Eliot wrote long ago. Often we believe, because we love an animal very much, that we are loved in return. This usually applies to companion dogs and cats, who are limited to one section in this chapter because such human–pet relationships are so common and universal.[1] But that our animal friends love us can be a dangerous assumption. Dale Lott's (2002) mother, who thought that she and her horse Smoky were great buddies, was killed when he suddenly threw himself backward so that the saddle horn was driven into her heart. Lott also describes a rancher in Idaho who raised a bull from a calf. Even when the animal was full-grown, he would let the man pet him and climb onto his back. Then one day the bull killed the man, mutilating his body and refusing to allow it to be removed from the corral. Lott writes that bison, for example, are "immune to our charm, sincerity, personal integrity and peaceful intentions," no matter what we may think. One man, who kept a few pet bison, was stunned one day when a young bull attacked him. The upward thrust of his horn into the man's belly and ribs was so strong that it chucked him over the fence where a veterinarian was able to save his life.

We cannot ever know if people and animals, even reptiles, can be best buddies.[2] The people may think they are, but their buddy may "think" otherwise, as the above examples indicate. The first four relationships described in this chapter about Elsa, the lion, mountain gorillas, olive baboons, and sociable whales do seem to depict true friendship. The animals are free to stay or leave the people they relate to, so there is equality between them. The second type of example includes horses and elephants who work for individual people. These animals and their human exploiters may have a good relationship, but it is not equitable. The animals must do what the humans expect and want. The same is true for the wolf Brenin and the hyrax Tsavo (and dogs), examples of the third type, but these animals, at least, were not expected to work for their keep. They did not try to escape from their close human buddies but were still subject to their humans' whims. The fourth and final type includes individuals who were subject to close human supervision by researchers devoted to teaching them to learn information that presumably exhibited their intelligence. These animals had no life of their own, although they were very close to their teachers who spent thousands of hours with them, drilling them on subjects important to people. But they were locked up at night when their work was done.

ELSA, THE LION, AND THE ADAMSONS

Joy Adamson's book *Born Free: A Lioness of Two Worlds* (2000) hit the reading world in 1960 like a bombshell. Millions bought or read the book. People leafing through it gaped at the photographs of full-grown Elsa flopped on a camp cot beside George, Joy's husband, or giving Joy a big smooching kiss. How could this be?

Elsa and her two sisters had been orphaned when their mother, a man-eater, had been hunted down and shot. George Adamson was a Game Warden of the Northern Frontier Province in Kenya, who agreed that he and Joy would try to raise them by hand. They were so successful with their efforts that the three cubs were soon rushing around the house and garden, knocking over furniture, ripping up cushions, and stalking each other and unsuspecting people. After being fed for twelve weeks largely on milk, they were given bits of meat as well. Elsa was smaller than her sisters and unable to get her fair share, so Joy took to feeding her on her lap. This was the beginning of their deep bond. Elsa showed her contentment by rolling her head from side to side and closing her eyes. She would massage Joy's legs with her front paws, as cats do, and suck her thumbs. Eventually, the threesome became so difficult to handle that the Adamsons sent two of the cubs to the Rotterdam Zoo. They could not bear to part with Elsa, though.

Elsa continued to grow, accompanied on forays into the bush or when resting by a young African lad hired to be with her. At tea-time, the Adamsons took her on another walk during which she climbed trees, stalked antelope (unsuccessfully), or investigated new creatures such as turtles, which she rolled about. In the evening, Joy sat with her in her enclosure while she ate, scooping out the marrow from bones that Elsa licked from her fingers, leaning her heavy body against her friend. Then Joy would play with Elsa, read, or sketch her. She writes "These evenings were our most intimate time, and I believe that her love for us was mostly fostered in these hours when, fed and happy, she could doze off with my thumb still in her mouth."

The Adamsons' aim was to have Elsa, when full-grown, return to the wild to live out her life there, something that had never been done before with a hand-reared cub. They prepared for this by taking her on a number of safaris into the barren country north of their house in Isiolo, where elephants, rhinoceros, and antelope were common. Elsa was quick to frighten and harry animals, but fortunately for them, unable to kill anything at first. At one point, George shot a waterbuck near her and as it fell, she grabbed it by the throat, which presumably gave her some idea of what killing meant. Gradually, she became used to eating wild animals, but if she were nervous, she still sucked Joy's thumb. Finally, they left Elsa in a wild area for a week and to their joy, when they returned to find out how she was getting on, her stomach was full. Although she was never able to join a lion pride, as these are closed to females not native to them, she did live successfully on her own, even producing cubs. Elsa continued to join, purr, and rub against her human friends whenever they visited her and announced their arrival by shooting off a rifle; she died prematurely in George's tent from a parasite infection.

MOUNTAIN GORILLAS AND DIAN FOSSEY

Surely the greatest love between wild animals and humans must be that between Dian Fossey and her gorillas. Many zoologists have spent much of their lives in the wild studying "their" species, but none gave as much of herself to them as did Fossey. She not only sat watching them in thin mountain air during long years of freezing rain and fog, but she also had to combat, year after year, the encroachment of poachers into the domain of the gorillas who would probably have wiped them out had she not fought them so aggressively. In the end, her efforts at protection probably cost her her life, as she was brutally murdered by an unknown assailant in her hut in 1985 (Mowat, 1987).

In her diary, Fossey writes that one of the outstanding moments of her life was on July 5, 1983, when she returned to the gorillas of group 5, her favorites, after an imposed absence from Africa of three years (Mowat, 1987). Would the gorillas remember her, she thought, as she climbed with her staff, for two long hours, up the mountain toward the group. When they located the animals, Fossey worked her way softly to within seven meters (23 ft) of them where she hunkered down and began making a series of soft rumbles like those made by contented gorillas. Old Effie, the nearest female whom Fossey had known since 1967, was chewing on a stalk of celery when she glanced over at the newcomer. She looked away, then looked quickly back, staring as if she could not believe her eyes. She tossed aside her celery and started toward her old friend. But Tuck, a younger female, got there first. She stopped right in front of Fossey, her weight resting on her arms, their faces several inches apart. They stared at each other for thirty or forty seconds. Fossey then lay down on a pile of vegetation, not knowing what else to do, while Tuck sniffed her head and neck, lay down beside her, and embraced her. Fossey wrote, "and embraced me … embraced me! … embraced me! GOD, she *did* remember!"

Tuck began crooning, and Fossey crooned back. Effie, who had arrived by now, also stared into Fossey's eyes, sniffed her, then piled on the two of them. By this time other gorillas in the dense foliage, who were aware of something going on, came forward, too. Four of them who had known Fossey also peered into her face before joining the group, "then settled down with long arms entwining all of us into one big, black, furry ball." They murmured as they crowded in, as if to say "Where the hell have you been? Is this really you?" Fossey was squished among the six excited gorillas, but euphoric. "I could have happily died right then and there and wished for nothing more on earth, simply because they had remembered," she wrote.

OLIVE BABOONS

Barbara Smuts (2001) spent every day, over two years, visiting and observing a baboon troop in Kenya. At first the animals fled when she approached them, but gradually they became used to her. In time, they accepted her as one of their own. Smuts describes resting in the shade of a tree with two of them, Alex leaning over to examine a colored stone she is holding before settling down against the tree trunk and Daphne acknowledging her presence with a friendly glance. A slight breeze breaks the stillness. Birds flit through the branches above. Soon, all of them have drifted off to sleep, safe among friends.

Smuts refers to this level of trust and familiarity, indeed affection, as "mutuality," which can occur between animals and people as well as within an animal community. It may develop between non-human individuals who share activities over time, such as play, sex, grooming, or joint activities (like hunting). Between an animal and a person, a bond is evident when the two have moved beyond merely understanding each other's usual behaviors and have developed a new language and culture particular to their own relationship. Such a bond need not imply any practical benefit to the two individuals, but is a commitment to the relationship "no matter what." Smuts writes, "Those of us who have experienced such relationships know that they are deeply rewarding. Indeed, for many people, they are the most fulfilling part of life."

FRIENDLY WHALES

Whale-watching vessels are ethically obliged to keep well back from whales lest they disturb and harass them. But what about whales who are attracted to people, or at least to their boats? Mary Lou Jones and Steven Swartz (1984) carried out research on gray whales (*Eschrichtius robustus*) in the breeding lagoons of Laguna San Ignacio in Baja, California, to determine the effect on them of human activity. Many female whales and their calves congregate there in a small area, so the Mexican government wanted to make sure that the animals were fully protected. At first, in 1975, a few whales were curious enough about boats to approach them, apparently interested in the noises made by their engines, which were at about the same frequency range as their own communications (Dahlheim et al., 1984). Boats idling or traveling slowly at about three knots an hour so attracted some whales that they hung around them for up to three hours, some leaving only when their engines were shut off. The whales avoided canoes, sailboats, and kayaks.

When whales approached their boat, people took to patting them, which the whales seemed to like. In 1982, Jones and Swartz personally had encounters with 200 such friendly whales during 70 days of their 97-day research season. In 1981, 26 of 28 excursion vessels had contacts with curious whales of both sexes and all ages, during which almost every one of the 700 passengers was able to "pet a whale." The researchers noted that although the whales were generally gentle and timid, they sometimes splashed their admirers or bumped up against their boat; six people had been thrown overboard by such collisions. The gray whale community seems to have forgotten the slaughters of the past by whaling boats, because their members were now offering friendship.

HORSES AND THEIR RIDERS

Friendship between a horse and a person can only begin when the horse is willing to allow the person within her flight distance, and to continue, she must be relaxed enough to allow him into her personal space around her body. This second imperative must be at the instigation of the horse, when she has become bold, curious, or lonely enough to approach the person of her own accord (Rees, 1997). This approach can be facilitated by bribes of food, but cannot be forced. Once the person is accepted close to the horse, he can offer the animal signs of friendship she understands – grooming, scratching, and rubbing. Friendship will also flourish when she is rewarded for her behavior by praise and encouragement rather than by punishment for her mistakes. One must always respect a horse in order to build trust with her or him.

Once a person is welcomed into a horse's personal space, he becomes, in her eyes, part of her social system. She will accept him as leader, do what he asks, and tolerate almost anything required of her in the way of training. She is indeed a social animal. Lucy Rees notes, "A befriended horse works hard for praise, and his joy and delight in pleasing his trainer are wonderful to see." Sadly, friendship between a person and a horse virtually always means one taking advantage of the other by sitting on her and bossing her about. Horses are often magnanimous enough to overlook this inequality and able to respond to requests for various commands rather than submitting to them.

English woman Barbara Woodhouse (1954), in her book *Talking to Animals 'The Woodhouse Way,'* describes her close bond with a 27-year-old horse she bought, called Tommy. She wanted to revive the worn-out spirit of this emaciated, sway-backed animal. By constant repetition and reward, she was able to teach him to walk on his hind legs, climb a ladder, and count. She played games with him, such as cowboys and Indians – he would race with her astride his back to escape from imaginary enemies and then lie down so she could hide behind him and return fire. She writes that Tommy did not know what game they were playing, but he loved working with her so much that he was willing to do whatever she wanted. They shared a wonderful friendship that brought pleasure into both their lives.

Recently, sociology professor Colleen Dell from the University of Saskatchewan has been working with the "spiritual bond between horses and humans" to help heal aboriginal youths who have problems with solvent abuse. Her approach, called equine-assisted learning, is approved by the Canadian Youth Solvent Addiction Committee (http://www.pimatisiwin.com), which is a world leader in this field. By learning to care for and ride these non-judgmental animals, the youths begin to gain self-respect.

ELEPHANTS AND MAHOUTS

Surely the closest animal–human friendships going back as far as 5000 years ago have been between mahouts and elephants (Hart and Sundar, 2000). In East Asia, elephants (*Elephas maximus*) guided by mahouts are still used in forestry; the animals are strong enough to haul logs and, compared to bulldozers that last at most ten years, economical because they begin work at about 20 years old, retire 40 years later, work without pay, and do not need to be constantly refueled. In addition, they do less damage to the environment (Chadwick, 1992).

The elephants have to work for a living but so do their mahouts, who in some cases remain with and care for the same elephant for their joint lifetimes. Douglas Chadwick (1992) visited the Mudumalai Sanctuary Elephant Camp in September 1989, just after logging operations had shut down for three months because of monsoon rains. During this season of respite, many mahouts accompanied their elephants to the river twice a day, dawn and mid-afternoon, to scrub them down as they lolled in the water, an activity that bonded the two because the elephants so enjoyed it. Washing them thoroughly freed the animals' skin from ticks, mites, lice, and leeches, and cleansed any cuts or scrapes to prevent infection. For breakfast, the mahouts cooked them cakes of rough wheat and molasses. After their second bath, they were hobbled by tying their front feet loosely together to restrain their wanderings, then let loose in the forest to forage and sleep during the night. The day before Chadwick arrived, the mahouts had thrown a party for their charges to thank them for their months of labor. They had painted the elephants' foreheads before giving them a feast of rice, fruits, and sweets bought with their own earnings. The men told Chadwick about a mahout who had ridden his bull to the local tavern many evenings, where he would buy a bottle of whiskey for the elephant and several for himself. When he keeled over from too much drink, the bull picked him up as if he were a log, wrapping his trunk around the mahout's body and placing him on his two huge tusks. Then he carried him home, deposited him on his doorstep, and waited for someone to come and pull him indoors before returning to his corral.

In Thailand where elephants also work in forestry, mahouts nowadays are less devoted to their charges than were their fathers and grandfathers, who sometimes slept in the bush with them (a challenge because elephants only sleep three or four hours at night and can travel surprisingly far when hobbled). The bond between elephant and mahout now is weaker because many of the men ride home in the evening on motorcycles to watch television and enjoy village life. Because they spend less time with their charges, the mahouts are less able to read the behavior of their elephants, and a number of men have been attacked or killed by them.

WOLF BRENIN AND MARK ROWLANDS

Many people think that you cannot be fast friends with a wolf, but Mark Rowlands (2009) found this to be untrue. He bought Brenin when he was six weeks old and, except for a quarantine period of six months when they moved from Alabama to Ireland, they were together every day for eleven years until Brenin died. Their day began when the wolf licked Rowlands in the face to waken him. Because Rowlands learned that wolves get bored very, very quickly and, if left alone, will rip all the furniture to shreds along with carpets and curtains, scenting them all with urine, Brenin accompanied him to the college where, as a professor, he lectured on philosophy to a class while Brenin mostly lay curled in the corner. Rarely, the wolf roamed about to try to wrestle some nervous student's lunch from his backpack, but he was not interested in the students themselves, or in any person but Mark. He ignored small dogs too, but would fight big dogs until Rowlands, who was very strong himself, physically forced him to stop. The two had frequent cuddles on the sofa at Brenin's instigation, chased each other in play, and ran side by side for miles every day for exercise. They went shopping together, although Brenin stayed in the van when Rowlands made brief forays into stores to buy provisions. They did everything as a pair.

A year before he died, Brenin got an infection in his anal glands, which Rowlands had to rinse out and inject with an antibacterial solution every two hours, night and day, to save his life. Rowlands hated this task as much as Brenin hated it and suffered from being treated. But the treatments made the professor realize how much he loved the wolf – not *eros*, erotic love; not *agape*, the impersonal love of God and humanity; but *philia*, the love of family or the pack. He loved Brenin as a brother, and undoubtedly Brenin doted on him in return.

WOLF PACK AND SHAUN ELLIS

As he describes in his book *The Man Who Lives with Wolves* (2009), Shaun Ellis gave a large part of his life to packs of wolves rather than to a single wolf such as Brenin. While growing up in England, he grew to love the natural world and eventually wolves, although there were no longer wild wolves in England. He flew to the Rocky Mountain area of Idaho, where he teamed up with Nez Percé natives, to study wolves in the wild. This evolved into him patiently stalking and then being accepted into a pack of four wolves (two males and two females, with the active breeder Miss Grumpy) over a two-year period, during which he never returned to the base camp at all. Ellis managed to insinuate himself into the group by being submissive to all the other members, in effect being the omega animal. He subsisted on fish and small game he snared, and eventually on chunks of deer meat brought to him by the pack. They called to each other in howls when they were apart, and when the animals returned from a hunt, Ellis and the others all licked each other excitedly around the mouth: "I was part of the pack, the wolves had accepted me, protected me, fed me." He was never part of the hunt itself, of course, because he was too slow and cumbersome, nor could he regurgitate food for the hungry cubs when they nibbled at his face.

Ellis hated to leave the pack when he returned to the camp to become a man again, but his first shower felt magnificent and the first human food he ate, a half jar of honey, delectable. He had learned an incredible amount about wolf behavior, which interested wolf biologists, but they were angry with him for risking his life and perhaps the life of the pack members who might now approach other people in friendship and be shot. Ellis has founded a Wolf Pack Foundation in England through which he offers advice to those interested and produces successful television programs about wolves.

HYRAX TSAVO AND THE FOSTERS

Human beings keep a huge variety of wild creatures in their care, no matter how unsatisfactory a life it means for their charge. Some animals seem happy enough, though, and some require a minimum of care. Such an animal was Tsavo, a lovable bush hyrax (*Heterohyrax brucei*) owned by my former classmate biologist Bristol Foster (1991), whom he had rescued in Kenya as an infant and brought to his home in British Columbia. Tsavo loved all the members of the family, following them about in the house or garden, and cuddling for warmth and companionship on their necks. In the wild, hyrax defecate on one spot, so it was easy to train Tsavo to use the toilet. Visitors had to be reminded to always leave the lid up so that Tsavo could be accommodated.

DOGS

The best-known example of attachment of a dog for his human companion is Bobby, a young Skye terrier who lived in Edinburgh, Scotland, with his great buddy Jock Gray (Coren, 2008). The pair would often lunch in a coffee house that stood near Greyfriars Church. When Gray died in 1858, he was buried in the Greyfriars churchyard. Bobby stayed in the churchyard after the funeral service was over, the grave closed and the mourners departed. In fact, he stayed by the grave for the rest of his life, 14 years, apparently waiting for his best friend to return. He is memorialized there by a small statue of the little dog erected in 1873, and by the name of the inn, now known as Greyfriars Bobby Inn.

Dogs are, in effect, a human invention because they have been bred for thousands of generations according to human specifications. Dogs may bond with one person in a family (most likely for a male dog), or with all family members (especially for a female dog [Coren, 2008]). Bonds are strengthened when a dog is stroked and petted, behaviors which release hormones such as oxytocin into the blood in both participants; people who live with dogs have lower blood pressure and reduced cholesterol levels on average than people without dogs in their home. During the catastrophic hurricane that flooded New Orleans in 2005, many people preferred to face death rather than be rescued and have to leave behind their beloved pet.

Dogs are a boon to prisoners serving long sentences for their crimes. In the Lansing Correctional Center in Kansas, under the Safe Harbor Prison Dog Program, about 100 inmates are training dogs who would have been facing death row themselves had they not been reprieved for the program (Riedel, 2006). Over some weeks, the men teach each dog basic commands so that they have a chance of being adopted, like the 1000 dogs trained before them. The trainers love the companionship and are less depressed than usual while working with the dogs, and the dogs love the attention, playing with their humans often while wearing the leashes, collars, or sweaters their friends have made for them.

CHIMPANZEES WASHOE, NIM, AND TRAVIS
AND THEIR MINDERS

Roger Fouts (1997) grew up on a small Californian farm where he learned to love animals. For graduate studies, he was challenged to work with Washoe, a young female chimpanzee, to see if he could teach her American Sign Language. It was known already that chimpanzees could not master human languages because of the anatomy of their vocal equipment. Fouts and his colleagues never spoke around Washoe so she would not realize there were other ways to communicate besides with gestures. Gradually, he taught her to make some American Sign Language signs, although there was always controversy about whether Washoe was just imitating her caretakers or actually taking part in language. He also taught her to eat with a knife and fork, leaf through magazines to see the pictures, and paint with brushes or with her fingers. After years of togetherness, Fouts was no longer able to care for his charge and was forced, to his horror, to put her into a crowded chimpanzee colony with few amenities. At the time, there were no facilities on the whole American continent where apes would be treated humanely and with respect. Fouts had grown to love Washoe and the other chimpanzees with whom he came in contact, and his love seemed to be returned. He could not bear that chimpanzees should be treated so badly. He writes that Washoe was his chimpanzee sister, and that since they had first met, "Washoe's chimpanzee family and my human family had become kin."[3]

Because of his love for Washoe and her chimpanzee friends and his shame for how such wonderful animals were treated by research institutions, Fouts spent ten years fund-raising, eight years designing, and two years building his dream place in the state of Washington: the Chimpanzee and Human Communication Institute. All the staff and the animals were thrilled when it opened in 1993, comprising large indoor spaces, a kitchen, and an expansive outdoor area, three stories high, bordered by mesh fencing. Washoe, who was now 28 years old, could spend her days chasing other chimpanzees, swinging high to the ceiling, or conversing in sign language with her human friends. Fouts has radically changed the future of many chimpanzees no longer wanted for research purposes, but with no other place to go were it not for his Institute.

People's efforts to humanize chimpanzees almost always end badly. One famous example was Nim Chimpsky, playfully misnamed after Noam Chomsky, who argued that human language was an orderly system of symbols governed by a set of unknown rules and impossible for any other species (Hess, 2008). Washoe had shown that an animal could learn American Sign Language, but Nim, it was hoped, would be able to use language as people do, rather than merely imitating the gestures of his trainer.

Nim was dragooned into being an experimental animal when he was yanked from his mother's breast aged ten days, and forced to begin training when two months old (Hess, 2008). He was raised for two years by Stephanie LaFarge, a psychologist with the American Society for the Prevention of Cruelty to Animals, along with her own children, dressed like a child, fed human food, given red wine, and successfully taught to speak with his hands. However, he was a handful – immensely strong although no bigger than a toddler, able to pick locks and escape from his family, and all too willing to trash his surroundings. Sometimes he bit people. When he was still young, LaFarge had to give him up.

Experts decided that although Nim could sign, he did not really have a language. Variety is the spice of life, but perhaps the 60 different teachers over four years with whom he had worked were too many for him (Tremain, 1982). Nim was removed from his family, put into a cage with screaming animals he had never seen before (i.e. chimpanzees), sold to a research facility, and finally moved to the Black Beauty Ranch animal sanctuary in Texas run by Cleveland Amory. When LaFarge visited him there many years after they had parted, he grabbed her when she entered his cage and roughed her up. He remembered that she had abandoned him and wanted her to know this, but he did not kill her as he could have. He died of a massive heart attack at the early age of 26.[4]

More recently, a chimpanzee called Travis, who also thought he was a human being, came to a violent end (Wente, 2009). He had been a celebrity in his youth, starring in B-grade TV movies and shilling for Old Navy and Coca-Cola. When he was washed up as an entertainer, he lived with his long-time friend, Sandra Herold, in Connecticut. She fed him fine food and wine, and he brushed her hair every evening. When she went out, he kissed her good-bye. However, in February 2009, he escaped from their house. When she and a woman friend tried to recapture him, he attacked the friend, whom he may have thought was a threat or a rival for Ms Herold's affection. The friend was badly injured so Herold tried to stop Travis's attack by stabbing him with a knife, then clubbing him with a shovel. When help arrived, Travis was shot and injured by the police. His blood trail led back to the house where he was found dead in his bedroom.

ALEX, THE GRAY AFRICAN PARROT, AND IRENE PEPPERBERG

Irene Pepperberg (Pepperberg, 2008) did her best *not* to become a fast friend of the gray African parrot (*Psittacus erithacus*) she bought one June day in 1977. There were eight of these birds for sale at a pet shop, but rather than pick one who appealed to her, she asked the salesman to choose. She did not want to be accused later of unscientific bias in her future studies of the bird's intelligence. For this reason, she also did not keep him and his cage in her home, but rather in her lab at the university. Alex was to be a one-pound colleague with gray feathers and a red tail; together they would work to discover how intelligent he was in tasks set by Pepperberg. They spent many thousands of hours together, day after day, year after year, for 30 years. How could they not become best buddies? She taught him to speak in clear English; if another bird slurred his words, Alex admonished him to "Speak better." She trained him to count up to seven, learn colors and textures, and speak in phrases. During their myriad of sessions together, Pepperberg discovered that he understood concepts such as bigger, smaller, more, fewer, and none. He was capable of thought and intention. Many television appearances and printed stories made him world famous. When Alex died of an infection about twenty years prematurely, almost his last words to Pepperberg before she left him in his cage for the night were, "You be good. I love you." She answered, "I love you, too." Pepperberg was devastated by his death. She will carry on her scientific research with other birds on the vast, almost unbelievable ability of the "bird brain," but her friendships with them will never be the same.

TIKO, THE AMAZON PARROT, AND JOANNA BURGER

Tiko was a red-lored Amazon parrot (*Amazona autumnalis*) lucky enough, when he was thirty years old and in his prime, to come to live with ornithologist Joanna Burger, who teaches animal behavior at Rutgers University. Burger was not interested in teaching Tiko as her colleague Irene Pepperberg had been for Alex, but she did want to observe his behavior and be his friend. You cannot rush a parrot, though, as Burger explains in her book, *The Parrot Who Owns Me* (2001). She took pains never to invade Tiko's space unless he wanted her to do so. She writes, "Parrots want to make their own friends at their own speed; pushing them provokes fear or aggression." He was often moody at first, but then he began to fit into family life: watching Burger as she rode her exercise bike; finding chocolates hidden for him by Mike, Joanna's husband; allowing his new acquaintances to gently scratch his head; and flying from room to room once he had regained his strength from being caged too long. He is tame, but not domesticated.

Tiko had bonded earlier with two women and, since he was born in captivity, he had become imprinted on humans. He fell in love with

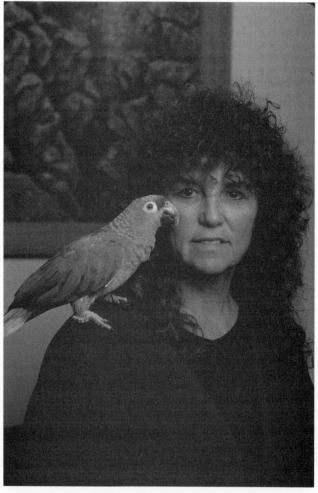

Figure 11. Joanna Burger with Tiko, the Amazon parrot.
© Joanna Burger

and began courting Joanna Burger five years after he had moved into her house. He became the alpha parrot of the household, Joanna his mate, and Mike an imposter of whom he was intensely jealous. When she woke each morning, he softly preened her finger tips with his bill and tongue, gently removing stray bits of skin and trimming her nails. He watched TV with his people (he and Mike especially liked reruns of *Cheers* and *Friends*) but refused to allow Mike to touch Joanna, or Joanna to address Mike in a sentimental voice. He even chose a place for the nest he and Joanna would share – under the credenza, which was only two inches above the floor. He would peek out from this cramped space, fixing Joanna with his eyes, and moaning enticingly. Sometimes he rushed out to her toes and preened them frantically before scooting back to his nest. Joanna proved an unwilling consort, though, and refused ever to join him there.

Parrots are intensely social. Without company, they will often lapse into depression, stop eating, stop playing, and become morose or even angry. Their loneliness leads them to excessive preening and to pulling out their feathers, leaving patches of bare skin. Joanna Burger saved Tiko from this fate. He is now in his fifties, sure of himself and of his close friendship with Joanna. He could live to be seventy. She must go on field trips for her scientific research, but she begins to worry about him after she has been away for three weeks or so. He continues to court her each spring, more frantically now than ever, with new nesting sites such as under the bedroom dresser, but these also are unsuccessful in attracting his finicky Joanna to nest with him. Even so, the woman and the parrot will surely remain fast friends for as long as they live.

Although parrots give their human companions great pleasure, the trade in these birds is devastating natural populations. In a recent five-year span, more than 4.2 million parrots were legally exported from their native lands to become the pets of humans (Burger, 2001). In addition, many birds are captured illegally; each year about 150,000 parrots are smuggled into the United States across the Mexican border. Methods to collect these birds in South America are horrendous, including nooses set among wild fruit that parrots eat, and cutting down trees in which parrots are nesting. During the smuggling operation itself, many parrots die of asphyxiation or trauma. How terrible that a possible friendship between a bird and a person should begin in such a horrific way.

Undoubtedly many millions of people have developed deep friendships with animals that have brightened their existence. It would be wonderful if these men and women and others would work together to improve the lives of all creatures so that such relationships could be extended. Then there would be less cruelty to animals through research experiments, hunting, fishing, rodeos, circuses with animal acts, and factory farms. Friendships could flourish as never before.

References

A Murder of Crows. 2009, Oct 10. TV program, Canadian Broadcasting Corporation.

Abegglen, J-J. 1985. *On Socialization in Hamadryas Baboons*. Cranbury, NJ: Associated University Presses.

Adamson, G. 1986. *My Pride and Joy: An Autobiography*. London: Collins Harvill.

Adamson, J. 2000 [1960]. *Born Free: A Lioness of Two Worlds*. New York: Pantheon Books.

Adkins-Regan, E. and M. Tomaszycki. 2007. Monogamy on the fast track. *Biology Letters*, **3**(6), 617–619.

Ardrey, R. 1961. *African Genesis: A Personal Investigation into the Animal Origins and Nature of Man*. New York: Atheneum.

Ardrey, R. 1966. *The Territorial Imperative: A Personal Inquiry into the Animal Origins of Property and Nations*. New York: Atheneum.

Ashworth, W. 1992. *Bears: Their Life and Behavior*. New York: Crown Publishers.

Bagemihl, B. 1999. *Biological Exuberance: Animal Homosexuality and Natural Diversity*. New York: St. Martin's Press.

Barrett, L. and S. P. Henzi. 2002. Constraints on relationship formation among female primates. *Behaviour*, **139**, 263–289.

Bartlett, T. Q. 2007. The Hylobatidae: Small apes of Asia. In C. J. Campbell, A. Fuentes, K. C. Mackinnon, M. Panger, and S. K. Bearder, eds. *Primates in Perspective*, 274–289. New York: Oxford University Press.

Bartlett, T. Q. 2009. *The Gibbons of Khao Yai: Seasonal Variation in Behavior and Ecology*. Upper Saddle River, NJ: Pearson Prentice Hall.

Barton, R. 1985. Grooming site preferences in primates and their functional implications. *International Journal of Primatology*, **6**(5), 519–532.

Bekoff, M. 2002. *Minding Animals: Awareness, Emotions, and Heart*. New York: Oxford University Press.

Bekoff, M. 2004. Coyotes: Clever tricksters, protean predators. In *Encyclopedia of Animal Behavior*, 447–451. Santa Barbara, CA: Greenwood Press.

Bekoff, M. 2007. *The Emotional Lives of Animals*. Novato, CA: New World Library.

Bentsen, C. 1989. *Maasai Days*. New York: Summit.

Bertram, B. 1978. *Pride of Lions*. London: Dent and Sons.

Blumstein, D. T. 2000. The evolution of infanticide in rodents: A comparative analysis. In C. P. van Schaik and C. H. Janson, eds. *Infanticide by Males and its Implications*, 178–197. Cambridge, UK: Cambridge University Press.

Boccia, M. L., M. Reite, and M. Laudenslager. 1989. On the physiology of grooming in a pigtail macaque. *Physiology and Behavior*, **45**, 667–670.

Boesch, C. 2002. Behavioural diversity in *Pan*. In C. Boesch, G. Hohmann, and L. F. Marchant, eds. *Behavioural Diversity in Chimpanzees and Bonobos*, 1–8. Cambridge, UK: Cambridge University Press.

Boesch, C. and H. Boesch-Achermann. 2000. *The Chimpanzees of the Taï Forest: Behavioural Ecology and Evolution*. Oxford, UK: Oxford University Press.

Boinski, S., K. Sughrue, L. Selvaggi, R. Quatrone, M. Henry, and S. Cropp. 2002. An expanded test of the ecological model of primate social evolution: Competitive regimes and female bonding in three species of squirrel monkeys (*Saimiri oerstedii, S. boliviensis*, and *S. sciurus*). *Behaviour*, **139**, 227–261.

Bonobo Conservation Initiative, 2006. http://www.bonobo.org

Bonobos: A Matriarchal Society. 2006. http://www.pacificviews.org/weblog/archives/002092.html

Broadminded robins. 2002, Mar 21. *Globe and Mail* (Toronto), A22.

Brockelman, W. Y., U. Reichard, U. Treesucon, and J. J. Raemaekers. 1998. Dispersal, pair formation and social structure in gibbons (*Hylobates lar*). *Behavioral and Ecological Sociobiology*, **42**, 329–339.

Bullington, S. W. No date. The hissing cockroach, *Gromphadorhina portentosa* (Schaum). http://www.zoo-zoom.com/hissing_cockroach.htm

Burger, J. 2001. *The Parrot Who Owns Me: The Story of a Relationship*. New York: Villard.

Busch, R. H. 2007. *The Wolf Almanac: A Celebration of Wolves and their World*. Guilford, CT: Globe Pequot.

Buss, I. O. 1990. *Elephant Life: Fifteen Years of High Population Density*. Ames, IA: Iowa State University Press.

Byers, J. A. 2003. *Built for Speed: A Year in the Life of Pronghorn*. Cambridge, MA: Harvard University Press.

Bygott, J. D., B. C. R. Bertram, and J. P. Hanby. 1979. Male lions in large coalitions gain reproductive advantages. *Nature*, **282**, 839–841.

Cacioppo, J. and W. Patrick. 2008. *Loneliness: Human Nature and the Need for Social Connection*. New York: Norton.

Cameron, E. Z., T. H. Setsaas, and W. L. Linklater. 2009. Social bonds between unrelated females increase reproductive success in feral horses. *Proceedings of the National Academy of Sciences of the United States of America*, **106**, 33, 13,850–13,853.

CBS News http://www.cbsnews.com/stories/2009/01/02/assignment_america/main4696340.shtml

Chadwick, D. H. 1992. *The Fate of the Elephant*. Toronto: Key Porter Books.

Chance, M. 1956. Social behaviour of rhesus monkeys: Social structure of a colony of *Macaca mulatta*. *British Journal of Animal Behaviour*, **4**, 1–13.

Chapais, B. and P. Bélisle. 2003. Constraints on kin selection in primate groups. In B. Chapais and C. M. Berman, eds. *Kinship and Behavior in Primates*, 365–386. Oxford, UK: Oxford University Press.

Cheney, D. L. and R. M. Seyfarth. 1990. *How Monkeys See the World: Inside the Mind of Another Species*. Chicago: University of Chicago Press.

Cheney, D. L. and R. M. Seyfarth. 2007. *Baboon Metaphysics: The Evolution of a Social Mind*. Chicago: University of Chicago Press.

Clutton-Brock, T. 2007. *Meerkat Manor: Flower of the Kalahari*. London: Weidenfeld and Nicolson.

Clutton-Brock, T. H., F. E. Guinness, and S. D. Albon. 1982. *Red Deer: Behavior and Ecology of Two Sexes*. Chicago: University of Chicago Press.

Clutton-Brock, T. H., J. M. Pemberton, T. Coulson, I. R. Stevenson, and A. D. C. MacColl. 2004. The sheep of St Kilda. In T. H. Clutton-Brock and

J. Pemberton, eds. *Soay Sheep: Dynamics and Selection in an Island Population*, 17–51. Cambridge, UK: Cambridge University Press.

Connor, R. C. 1995. Impala allogrooming and the parcelling model of reciprocity. *Animal Behaviour*, **49**, 528–530.

Connor, R. C. and D. M. Peterson. 1994. *The Lives of Whales and Dolphins*. New York: Henry Holt.

Connor, R. C., R. A. Smolker, and A. F. Richards. 1992. Dolphin alliances and coalitions. In A. H. Harcourt and F. B. M. de Waal, eds. *Coalitions and Alliances in Humans and Other Animals*, 414–443. Oxford, UK: Oxford University Press.

Cords, M. 1997. Friendships, alliances, reciprocity and repair. In A. Whiten and R. W. Byne, eds. *Machiavellian Intelligence 11: Extensions and Evaluations*, 24–49. Cambridge, UK: Cambridge University Press.

Cords, M. 2002. Friendship among adult female blue monkeys (*Cercopithecus mitis*). *Behaviour*, **139**, 291–314.

Coren, S. 2008. *The Modern Dog: A Joyful Exploration of How We Live with Dogs Today*. New York: Free Press.

Coren, S. 2010, Jan 9. The evolution of heroism. *Globe and Mail* (Toronto), A15.

Côté, S. D., M. Festa-Bianchet, and F. Fournier. 1998. Life-history effects of chemical immobilization and radio collars in mountain goats. *Journal of Wildlife Management*, **62**, 745–752.

Craighead, F. C. Jr. and J. J. Craighead. 1972. Grizzly bear prehibernation and denning activities as determined by radio tracking. *Wildlife Monographs*, No. 32.

Dagg, A. I. 1998. Infanticide by male lions hypothesis: A fallacy influencing research into human behavior. *American Anthropologist*, **100**(4), 1–11.

Dagg, A. I. 2001. The infanticide hypothesis: A response to the response. *American Anthropologist*, **102**(4), 831–834.

Dagg, A. I. 2005. *"Love of Shopping is Not a Gene": Problems with Darwinian Psychology*. Montreal: Black Rose Press.

Dagg, A. I. 2006. *Pursuing Giraffe: A 1950s Adventure*. Waterloo, ON: Wilfrid Laurier University Press.

Dagg, A. I. 2008. Blame and shame? How can we reduce unproductive animal experimentation? In J. Castricano, ed. *Animal Subjects: An Ethical Reader in a Posthuman World*, 271–284. Waterloo, ON: Wilfrid Laurier University Press.

Dahlheim, M. E., H. D. Fisher, and J. D. Schempp. 1984. Sound production by the gray whale and ambient noise levels in Laguna San Ignacio, Baja California Sur, Mexico. In M. L. Jones, Steven L. Swartz, and S. Leatherwood, eds. 1984. *The Gray Whale: Eschrichtius robustus*, 511–541. Orlando, FL: Academic Press.

Darling, F. F. 1969 [1937]. *A Herd of Red Deer: A Study in Animal Behaviour*. London: Oxford University Press.

DeNault, L. K. and D. A. McFarlane. 1995. Reciprocal altruism between male vampire bats, *Desmodus rotundus*. *Animal Behaviour*, **49**, 855–856.

de Waal, F. 1997. *Bonobo: The Forgotten Ape*. Berkeley, CA: University of California Press.

de Waal, F. 2005. *Our Inner Ape: A Leading Primatologist Explains Why We Are Who We Are*. New York: Riverhead Books.

de Waal, F. 2008. Foreword to behavioral study section. In Furuichi, T. and J. Thompson, eds. *The Bonobos: Behavior, Ecology, and Conservation*, 11–14. New York: Springer.

Digby, L. 2000. Infanticide by female mammals: Implications for the evolution of social systems. In C. P. van Schaik and C. H. Janson, eds. *Infanticide by Males and its Implications*, 423–446. Cambridge, UK: Cambridge University Press.

Dobie, J. F. 1955. *The Mustangs*. London: Hammond, Hammond and Co.

Douglas, C. and P. Rowlinson. 2009, Jan 28. Exploring stock managers' perceptions of the human–animal relationship on dairy farms and an association with milk production. *Anthrozoos*, Berg Publishing on the web.

Dower, L. 1998. Other senses. In M. Tobias and K. Solisti-Mattelon, eds. *Kinship with Animals*, 259–264. Hillsboro, OR: Beyond Words Publishing.

Dunbar, R. I. M. 1983. Relationships and social structure in gelada and hamadryas baboons. In R. A. Hinde, ed. *Primate Social Relationships: An Integrated Approach*, 299–307. Sunderland, MA: Sinauer Associates.

Dunbar, R. I. M. 1991. Functional significance of social grooming in primates. *Folia Primatologica*, **57**, 121–131.

Dutcher, J. and J. Dutcher. 2002. *Wolves at our Door*. New York: Simon and Schuster.

Ellis, S. with P. Junor. 2009. *The Man who Lives with Wolves*. New York: Harmony Books.

Eltringham, S. K. 1999. *The Hippos: Natural History and Conservation*. London: Academic Press.

Emlen, S. T. 1982. The evolution of helping. 1. An ecological constraints model. *American Naturalist*, **119**(1), 29–39.

Engh, A. L., J. C. Beehner, T. J. Bergman, *et al.* 2006. Behavioural and hormonal responses to predation in female chacma baboons (*Papio hamadryas ursinus*). *Proceedings of the Royal Society B: Biological Sciences*, **273**, 707–712.

Fedigan, L. M. 1991. History of the Arashiyama West Japanese macaques in Texas. In L. M Fedigan and P. J. Asquith, eds. *The Monkeys of Arashiyama: Thirty-Five Years of Research in Japan and the West*, 54–73. Albany, NY: State University of New York Press.

Fedigan, L. M. and M. J. Baxter. 1984. Sex differences and social organization in free-ranging spider monkeys (*Ateles geoffroyi*). *Primates*, **25**(3), 279–294.

Feh, C. 1999. Alliances and reproductive success in Camargue stallions. *Animal Behaviour*, **57**(3), 705–713.

Feh, C. and J. de Mazières. 1993. Grooming at a preferred site reduces heart rate in horses. *Animal Behaviour*, **46**(6), 1191–1194.

Feldhake, G. 2005. *Hippos: Natural History and Conservation*. Stillwater, MN: Voyageur Press.

Fennessy, J. 2004. Ecology of desert-dwelling giraffe *Giraffa camelopardalis angolensis* in northwestern Namibia. PhD Thesis, University of Sydney. http://search.arrow.edu.au/main/results?subject=giraffe

Fernández, G. J. and J. C. Reboreda. 1995. Adjacent nesting and egg stealing between males of the greater rhea *Rhea americana. Journal of Avian Biology*, **26**, 321–324.

Festa-Bianchet, M. 1991. The social system of bighorn sheep: grouping patterns, kinship and female dominance rank. *Animal Behaviour*, **42**, 71–82.

Festa-Bianchet, M. and S. D. Côté. 2008. *Mountain Goats: Ecology, Behavior, and Conservation of an Alpine Ungulate*. Washington, DC: Island Press.

Feuerstein, N. and J. Terkel. 2008. Interrelationships of dogs (*Canis familiaris*) and cats (*Felis catus* L.) living under the same roof. *Applied Animal Behaviour Science*, **113**(1–3), 150–165.

Findley, T. 1998. *From Stone Orchard*. Toronto: Harper Flamingo.

Fossey, D. 1983. *Gorillas in the Mist*. Boston: Houghton Mifflin.

Foster, J. B. 1987, Jul/Aug. Walking tall. *Equinox*, **7**, 24–34.

Foster, J. B. 1991, Mar/Apr. Warming up to the hyrax. *International Wildlife*, **21**, 49–52.

Foster, J. B. and A. I. Dagg. 1972. Notes on the biology of the giraffe. *East African Wildlife Journal*, **10**, 1–16.

Fournier, F. and M. Festa-Bianchet. 1995. Social dominance in adult female mountain goats. *Animal Behaviour*, **49**, 1449–1459.

Fouts, R. with S.T. Mills. 1997. *Next of Kin: My Conversations with Chimpanzees*. New York: HarperCollins.

Fuentes, A. 2002. Patterns and trends in primate pair bonds. *International Journal of Primatology*, **23**(5), 953–978.

Furuichi, T. and J. Thompson. 2008. Introduction. In T. Furuichi and J. Thompson, eds. *The Bonobos: Behavior, Ecology, and Conservation*, 1–4. New York: Springer.

Geist, V. 1971. *Mountain Sheep: A Study in Behavior and Evolution*. Chicago: University of Chicago Press.

Geist, V. and R. Petocz. 1977. Bighorn sheep in winter: Do rams maximize reproductive fitness by spatial and habitat segregation from ewes? *Canadian Journal of Zoology*, **55**, 1802–1810.

Geist, V. and F. Walther, eds. 1974. *The Behaviour of Ungulates and its Relation to Management*. Morges, Switzerland: International Union for Conservation of Nature and Natural Resources.

Ghiglieri, M.P. 1988. *East of the Mountains of the Moon: Chimpanzee Society in the African Rain Forest*. London: Collier Macmillan.

Gier, H.T. 1975. Ecology and behavior of the coyote (*Canis latrans*). In M.W. Fox, ed. *The Wild Canids: Their Systematics, Behavioral Ecology and Evolution*, 247–262. New York: Van Nostrand Reinhold.

Goodall, J. 1986. *The Chimpanzees of Gombe: Patterns of Behavior*. Cambridge, MA: Belknap Press.

Goosen, C. 1987. Social grooming in primates. In G. Mitchell and J. Erwin, eds. *Behavior, Cognition, and Motivation*, 107–131. New York: Alan R. Liss.

Gordon, J. 1998. *Sperm Whales*. Stillwater, MN: Voyageur Press.

Griffin, A.S. 2008. Naked mole-rat. *Current Biology*, **18**(18), R844–R845.

Gunter, L. 2009, Jul 3. Don't pity the calves. *National Post* (Toronto), A14.

Hanby, J. 1982. *Lions Share: The Story of a Serengeti Pride*. Boston: Houghton Mifflin.

Hanson, T. 2008. *The Impenetrable Forest: My Gorilla Years in Uganda*. Warwick, NY: 1500 Books.

Harcourt, A.H. 1979. Social relationships among adult female mountain gorillas. *Animal Behaviour*, **27**, 251–264.

Harrison, C.J.O. 1965. Allopreening as agonistic behaviour. *Behaviour*, **24**, 161–208.

Hart, B.L. and L.A. Hart. 1992. Reciprocal allogrooming in impala, *Aepyceros melampus*. *Animal Behaviour*, **44**, 1073–1083.

Hart, B.L., L.A. Hart, M.S. Mooring, and R. Olubayo. 1992. Biological basis of grooming behaviour in antelope: The body-size, vigilance and habitat principles. *Animal Behaviour*, **44**, 615–631.

Hart, D. and R.W. Sussman. 2005. *Man the Hunted: Primates, Predators, and Human Evolution*. New York: Westview Press.

Hart, L. and Sundar. 2000. Family traditions for mahouts of Asian elephants. *Anthrozoos: A Multidisciplinary Journal of the Interactions of People and Animals*, **13**(1), 34–42.

Hatkoff, A. 2009. *The Inner World of Farm Animals: Their Amazing Social, Emotional, and Intellectual Capacities*. New York: Stewart, Tabori, and Chang.

Hearne, V. 2000. *Adam's Task: Calling Animals by Name*. New York: Akadine Press.

Heinrich, B. 2004. *The Geese of Beaver Bog*. New York: HarperCollins.

Henzi, S.P. and L. Barrett. 1999. The value of grooming to female primates. *Primates*, **40**(1), 47–59.

Henzi, S.P. and A. MacDonald. 1986, Sep/Oct. A baboon among goats. *African Wildlife*, 117.

Hess, E. 2008. *Nim Chimpsky: The Chimp who Would be Human*. New York: Bantam Dell.

Hill, D. A. 2004. The effects of demographic variation on kinship structure and behavior in Cercopithecines. In B. Chapais and C. M. Berman, eds. *Kinship and Behavior in Primates*, 132–150. Oxford, UK: Oxford University Press.

Hillegass, M. A., J. M. Waterman, and J. D. Roth. 2008. The influence of sex and sociality on parasite loads in an African ground squirrel. *Behavioral Ecology*, **19**(5), 1006–1011.

Hirotani, A. 1990. Social organization of reindeer (*Rangifer tarandus*), with special reference to relationships among females. *Canadian Journal of Zoology*, **68**, 743–749.

Hohmann, G., U. Gerloff, D. Tautz, and B. Fruth. 1999. Social bonds and genetic ties: kinship, association and affiliation in a community of bonobos (*Pan paniscus*). *Behaviour*, **136**, 1219–1235.

House, J. S., K. R. Landis, and D. Umberson. 1988. Social relationships and health. *Science*, **241**(4865), 540–545.

Hoyt, E. 1990. *Orca: The Whale Called Killer*. Toronto: Camden House.

Hrdy, S. B. 1977. *The Langurs of Abu: Female and Male Strategies of Reproduction*. Cambridge, MA: Harvard University Press.

Hrdy, S. B. 2009. *Mother and Others: The Evolutionary Origins of Mutual Understanding*. Cambridge, MA: Harvard University Press.

Huber, R. and M. Martys. 1993. Male-male pairs in greylag geese (*Anser anser*). *Journal of Ornithology*, **134**, 155–164.

Huchard, E., A. Alvergne, D. Fejan, *et al*. 2010. More than friends? Behavioural and genetic aspects of heterosexual associations in wild chacma baboons. *Behavioral Ecology and Sociobiology*, **64**(5), 769–781.

Hudson, W. H. 1923. *Birds and Man*. New York: Knopf.

Huffman, M. A. 1990. Some socio-behavioral manifestations of old age. In T. Nishida, ed. *The Chimpanzees of the Mahale Mountains: Sexual and Life History Strategies*, 237–255. Tokyo: University of Tokyo Press.

Idani, G. 1991. Social relationships between immigrant and resident bonobo (*Pan paniscus*) females at Wamba. *Folia Primatologica*, **57**, 83–95.

Idani, G., N. Mwanza, H. Ihobe, *et al*. 2008. Changes in the status of bonobos, their habitat, and the situation of humans at Wamba in the Luo Scientific Reserve, Democratic Republic of Congo. In T. Furuichi and J. Thompson, eds. *The Bonobos: Behavior, Ecology, and Conservation*, 201–302. New York: Springer.

Ihobe, H. 1992. Male-male relationships among wild bonobos (*Pan paniscus*) at Wamba, Republic of Zaire. *Primates*, **33**(2), 163–179.

Imber, M. J. 1973. The food of grey-faced petrels (*Pterodroma macroptera gouldi* [Hutton]), with special reference to diurnal vertical migration of their prey. *Journal of Animal Ecology*, **42**, 645–662.

Imber, M. J. 1976. Breeding biology of the grey-faced petrel *Pterodroma macroptera gouldi*. *Ibis*, **118**, 51–64.

Innis, A. C. 1958. The behaviour of the giraffe, *Giraffa camelopardalis*, in the eastern Transvaal. *Proceedings of the Zoological Society of London*, **131**, 245–278.

Isbell, L. A. and T. P. Young. 2002. Ecological models of female social relationships in primates: Similarities, disparities, and some directions for future clarity. *Behaviour*, **139**, 177–202.

Janson, C. H. and C. P. van Schaik. 2000. The behavioral ecology of infanticide by males. In C. P. van Schaik and C. H. Janson, eds. *Infanticide by Males and its Implications*, 469–494. Cambridge, UK: Cambridge University Press.

Jarvis, J. U. M. 1981. Eusociality in a mammal: Cooperative breeding in naked mole-rat colonies. *Science*, **212**(4494), 571–573.

Johanson, D. C. 2009. *Lucy's Legacy*. New York: Harmony Books.

Jolly, A. 1966. *Lemur Behavior: A Madagascar Field Study*. Chicago: University of Chicago Press.

Jolly, A. 2004. *Lords and Lemurs: Mad Scientists, Kings with Spears, and the Survival of Diversity in Madagascar*. Boston: Houghton Mifflin.

Jones, M. L. and S. L. Swartz. 1984. Demography and phenology of gray whales and evaluation of whale-watching activities in Laguna San Ignacio, Baja California Sur, Mexico. In M. L. Jones, S. L. Swartz, and S. Leatherwood, eds. *The Gray Whale: Eschrichtius robustus*, 309–374. Orlando, FL: Academic Press.

Kano, T. 1992. *The Last Ape: Pygmy Chimpanzee Behavior and Ecology*. Stanford, CA: Stanford University Press.

Kappeler, P. M. 2000. Primate males: History and theory. In P. M. Kappeler, ed. *Primate Males: Causes and Consequences of Variation in Group Composition*, 3–7. Cambridge, UK: Cambridge University Press.

Kato, E. 1999. Effects of age, dominance, and seasonal changes on proximity relationships in female Japanese macaques (*Macaca fuscata*) in a free-ranging group at Katsuyama. *Primates*, **40**(2), 291–300.

Kawanaka, K. 1990. Alpha males' interactions and social skills. In T. Nishida, ed. *The Chimpanzees of the Mahale Mountains: Sexual and Life History Strategies*, 171–187. Tokyo: University of Tokyo Press.

Kays, R. 2003. Social polyandry and promiscuous mating in a primate-like carnivore: the kinkajou (*Potos flavus*). In U. H. Reichard and C. Boesch, eds. *Monogamy: Mating Strategies and Partnerships in Birds, Humans and Other Mammals*, 125–137. Cambridge, UK: Cambridge University Press.

Kendrick, K. M., A. P. da Costa, A. E. Leigh, M. R. Hinton, and J. W. Pierce. 2001. Sheep don't forget a face. *Nature*, **414**, 165–166.

Keverne, E. B., N. D. Martensz, and B. Tuite. 1989. Beta-endorphin concentrations in cerebrospinal fluid of monkeys are influenced by grooming relationships. *Psychoneuroendocrinology*, **14**(1–2), 155–161.

Kilham, B. [with E. Gray]. 2002. *Among the Bears: Raising Orphan Cubs in the Wild*. New York: Henry Holt.

Kilham, L. 1989. *The American Crow and the Common Raven*. College Station, TX: Texas A and M University Press.

King, S. 2009. *The Cheetah Orphans*. PBS. http://www.pbs.org/wnet/nature/cheetahs

Klingel, H. 1998. Observations on social organization and behaviour of African and Asiatic Wild Asses (*Equus africanus* and *Equus hemionus*). *Applied Animal Behaviour Science*, **60**(2–3), 103–113.

Knudtson, P. 1996. *Orca: Visions of the Killer Whale*. Vancouver: Greystone Books.

Korstjens, A. H., E. H. M. Sterck, and R. Noë. 2002. How adaptive or phylogenetically inert is primate social behaviour? A test with two sympatric colobines. *Behaviour*, **139**, 203–225.

Koyama, N. 1991. Grooming relationships in the Arashiyama group of Japanese monkeys. In L. M. Fedigan and P. J. Asquith, eds. *The Monkeys of Arashiyama: Thirty-five Years of Research in Japan and the West*, 211–226. Albany, NY: State University of New York Press.

Kruuk, H. 1972. *The Spotted Hyena: A Study of Predation and Social Behavior*. Chicago: University of Chicago Press.

Kudo, H. and R. I. M. Dunbar. 2001. Neocortex size and social network size in primates. *Animal Behaviour*, **62**, 711–722.

Kummer, H. 1968. *Social Organization of Hamadryas Baboons: A Field Study*. Chicago: University of Chicago Press.

Kummer, H. 1995. *In Quest of the Sacred Baboon: A Scientist's Journey*. Princeton, NJ: Princeton University Press.

Kuo, Z. Y. 1930. The genesis of the cat's responses to the rat. *Comparative Psychology*, **11**, 1–35.

Lehmann, J. and C. Boesch. 2008. Sexual differences in chimpanzee sociality. *International Journal of Primatology*, **29**, 65–81.

Leuthold, W. 1974. Observations on home range and social organization of lesser kudu, *Tragelaphus imberbis* (Blyth, 1869). In V. Geist and F. Walther, eds. *The Behaviour of Ungulates and its Relation to Management*, Vol 1, 206–234. Morges, Switzerland: International Union for Conservation of Nature and Natural Resources.

Lewis, S., G. Roberts, M. P. Harris, C. Prigmore, and S. Wanless. 2007. Fitness increases with partner and neighbour allopreening. *Biology Letters*, **3**(4), 386–389.

Linden, E. 1999. *The Parrot's Lament and Other True Tales of Animal Intrigue, Intelligence, and Ingenuity*. New York: Penguin Group.

Lorenz, K. 1952. *King Solomon's Ring: New Light on Animal Ways*. New York: Thomas Crowell.

Lorenz, K. 1991. *Here I am – Where Are You? The Behavior of the Greylag Goose*. New York: Harcourt Brace Jovanovich.

Lott, D. F. 2002. *American Bison: A Natural History*. Berkeley, CA: University of California Press.

Lusseau, D. 2007. Evidence for social role in a dolphin social network. *Evolutionary Ecology*, **21**, 357–366.

Lusseau, D., K. Schneider, O. J. Boisseau, *et al.* 2003. The bottlenose dolphin community of Doubtful Sound features a large proportion of long-lasting associations: Can geographic isolation explain this unique trait? *Behavioral Ecology and Sociobiology*, **54**, 396–405.

Lusseau, D., B. Wilson, P. S. Hammond, *et al.* 2006. Quantifying the influence of sociality on population structure in bottlenose dolphins. *Journal of Animal Ecology*, **75**, 14–24.

Maestripieri, D. 1993. Vigilance costs of allogrooming in macaque mothers. *American Naturalist* **141**(5), 744–753.

Malenky, R. K. and R. W. Wrangham. 1994. A quantitative comparison of terrestrial herbaceous food consumption by *Pan panicus* in the Lomako Forest, Zaire, and *Pan troglodytes* in the Kibale Forest, Uganda. *American Journal of Primatology*, **32**, 1–12.

Manson, J. H., C. D. Navarrete, J. B. Silk, and S. Perry. 2004. Time-matched grooming in female primates? New analyses from two species. *Animal Behaviour*, **67**, 493–500.

Maples, E. G., M. M. Haraway, and C. W. Hutto. 1989. Development of coordinated singing in a newly formed siamang pair (*Hylobates syndactylus*). *Zoo Biology*, **8**(4), 367–378.

Marzluff, J. M. and T. Angell. 2005. *In the Company of Crows and Ravens*. New Haven: Yale University Press.

Masson, J. 1997. *Dogs Never Lie about Love: Reflections on the Emotional World of Dogs*. New York: Crown Publishers.

Masson, J. M. 1999. *The Emperor's Embrace: The Evolution of Fatherhood*. New York: Washington Square Books.

Masson, J. M. 2003. *The Pig Who Sang to the Moon: The Emotional World of Farm Animals*. New York: Ballantine Books.

McCarthy, S. 2004. *Becoming Tiger: How Baby Animals Learn to Live in the Wild*. New York: HarperCollins.

Méndez-Cárdenas, M. G. and E. Zimmermann. 2009. Duetting – a mechanism to strengthen pair bonds in a dispersed pair-living primate (*Lepilemur edwardsi*)? *American Journal of Physical Anthropology*, **139**, 523–532.

Milius, S. 2003, Nov 1. Beast buddies: Do animals have friends? *Science News*, **164**, 282–284.

Mitani, M. 1986. Voiceprint identification and its application to sociological studies of wild Japanese monkeys (*Macaca fuscata yakui*). *Primates*, **27**(4), 397–412.

Mitchell, C. L., S. Boinski, and C. P. van Schaik. 1991. Competitive regimes and female bonding in two species of squirrel monkeys (*Saimiri oerstedi* and *S. sciureus*). *Behavioral Ecology and Sociobiology*, **28**, 55–60.

Mloszewski, M. J. 1983. *The Behavior and Ecology of the African Buffalo*. Cambridge, UK: Cambridge University Press.

Montgomery, S. 1991. *Walking with the Great Apes: Jane Goodall, Dian Fossey, Biruté Galdikas*. Boston: Houghton Mifflin.

Mooallem, J. 2010, April 4. Can animals be gay? *New York Times, Sunday Magazine*, MM26.

Mooring, M. S., A. A. McKenzie, and B. L. Hart. 1996. Role of sex and breeding status in grooming and total tick load of impala. *Behavioral Ecology and Sociobiology*, **39**(4), 259–266.

Mori, U. 1979a. Inter-unit relationships. In M. Kawai, ed. *Ecological and Sociological Studies of Gelada Baboons*, 83–92. Basel: S. Karger.

Mori, U. 1979b. Individual relationships within a unit. In M. Kawai, ed. *Ecological and Sociological Studies of Gelada Baboons*, 93–124. Basel: S. Karger.

Mori, U. 1979c. Development of sociability and social status. In M. Kawai, ed. *Ecological and Sociological Studies of Gelada Baboons*, 125–154. Basel: S. Karger.

Morin, P. 2006. *Honest Horses: Wild Horses in the Great Basin*. Reno, NV: University of Nevada Press.

Morris, D. 1967. *The Naked Ape: A Zoologist's Study of the Human Animal*. New York: McGraw-Hill.

Morris, D. 1988. *Horse Watching*. New York: Crown Publishers.

Morton, A. 2002. *Listening to Whales: What the Orcas have Taught us*. New York: Ballantine Books.

Moss, C. 1988. *Elephant Memories: Thirteen Years in the Life of an Elephant Family*. New York: William Morrow.

Moss, C. J. and J. H. Poole. 1983. Relationships and social structure of African elephants. In R. A. Hinde, ed. *Primate Social Relationships: An Integrated Approach*, 315–325. Sunderland, MA: Sinauer Associates.

Mowat, F. 1987. *Virunga: The Passion of Dian Fossey*. Toronto: McClelland and Stewart.

Müller-Schwarze, D. and L. Sun. 2003. *The Beaver: Natural History of a Wetlands Engineer*. Ithaca, NY: Comstock Publishing (Cornell University Press).

Nagel, S. 2004. *Mistress of the Elgin Marbles: A Biography of Mary Nisbet, Countess of Elgin*. New York: HarperCollins.

Nakagawa, N. 1992. Distribution of affiliative behaviors among adult females within a group of wild patas monkeys in a nonmating, nonbirth season. *International Journal of Primatology*, **13**(1), 73–96.

Nakamichi, M. 1991. Behavior of old females: Comparisons of Japanese monkeys in the Arashiyama East and West groups. In L. M. Fedigan and P. J. Asquith, eds. 1991. *The Monkeys of Arashiyama: Thirty-Five Years of Research in Japan and the West*, 175–193. Albany, NY: State University of New York Press.

Nakamichi, M. 2003. Age-related differences in social grooming among adult female Japanese monkeys (*Macaca fuscata*). *Primates*, **44**, 239–246.

Nakamichi, M. and N. Koyama. 1997. Social relationships among ring-tailed lemurs (*Lemur catta*) in two free-ranging troops at Berenty Reserve, Madagascar. *International Journal of Primatology*, **18**(1), 73–93.

Nakamichi, M. and K. Yamada. 2007. Long-term grooming partnerships between unrelated adult females in a free-ranging group of Japanese monkeys (*Macaca fuscata*). *American Journal of Primatology*, **69**, 652–663.

Neuhaus, P. and K. E. Ruckstuhl. 2002. The link between sexual dimorphism, activity budgets, and group cohesion: The case of the plains zebra (*Equus burchelli*). *Canadian Journal of Zoology*, **80**, 1437–1441.

Newton-Fisher, N. 2002. Relationships of male chimpanzees in the Budongo Forest, Uganda. In C. Boesch, G. Hohmann, and L. F. Marchant, eds. *Behavioural Diversity in Chimpanzees and Bonobos*, 125–137. Cambridge, UK: Cambridge University Press.

Nishida, T. 1990. A quarter century of research in the Mahale Mountains: An Overview. In T. Nishida, ed. *The Chimpanzees of the Mahale Mountains: Sexual and Life History Strategies*, 3–35. Tokyo: University of Tokyo Press.

Noë, R. 2006. Digging for the roots of trading. In P. M. Kappeler and C. P. van Schaik, eds. *Cooperation in Primates and Humans: Mechanisms and Evolution*, 233–261. Berlin: Springer.

Ogawa, H. 1995. Bridging behavior and other affiliative interactions among male Tibetan macaques (*Macaca thibetana*). *International Journal of Primatology*, **16**(5), 707–729.

Ohsawa, H. 1979. The local gelada population and environment of the Gich Area. In M. Kawai, ed. *Ecological and Sociological Studies of Gelada Baboons*, 3–45. Basel: S. Karger.

Olmert, M. D. 2009. *Made for Each Other: The Biology of the Human–Animal Bond*. Cambridge, MA: Da Capo Press.

Olson, S. 2006. Neanderthal Man. *Smithsonian Magazine, Science and Nature*, Oct. http://www.smithsonianmag.com/science-nature/neanderthal.html

Overdorff, D. J. 1998. Are *Eulemur* species pair-bonded? Social organization and mating strategies in *Eulemur fulvus rufus* from 1988–1995 in southeast Madagascar. *American Journal of Physical Anthropology*, **105**, 153–166.

Owens, M. and D. Owens. 2006. *Secrets of the Savanna: Twenty-three Years in the African Wilderness Unraveling the Mysteries of Elephants and People*. Boston: Houghton Mifflin.

Owen-Smith, N. 1974. The social system of the white rhinoceros. In V. Geist and F. R. Walther, eds. *The Behaviour of Ungulates and its Relation to Management*, 341–351. Morges, Switzerland: International Union for Conservation of Nature and Natural Resources.

Packer, C., D. A. Gilbert, A. E. Pusey, and S. J. O'Brieni. 1991. A molecular genetic analysis of kinship and cooperation in African lions. *Nature*, **351**, 562–565.

Packer, C. and A. E. Pusey. 1982. Cooperation and competition within coalitions of male lions: Kin selection or game theory? *Nature*, **296**, 740–742.

Palombit, R. A. 1996. Pair bonds in monogamous apes: A comparison of the siamang *Hylobates syndactylus* and the white-handed gibbon *Hylobates lar*. *Behaviour*, **133**, 321–356.

Palombit, R. A. 2000. Infanticide and the evolution of male–female bonds in animals. In C. P. van Schaik and C. H. Janson, eds. *Infanticide by Males and its Implications*, 239–268. Cambridge, UK: Cambridge University Press.

Palombit, R. A., R. M. Seyfarth and D. L. Cheney. 1997. The adaptive value of "friendships" to female baboons: experimental and observational evidence. *Animal Behaviour*, **54**, 599–614.

Paul, A., S. Preuschoft, and C. P. van Schaik. 2000. The other side of the coin: Infanticide and the evolution of affiliative male–infant interactions in Old World primates. In C. P. van Schaik and C. H. Janson, eds. *Infanticide by Males and its Implications*, 269–292. Cambridge, UK: Cambridge University Press.

Pepperberg, I. M. 2008. *Alex and Me*. New York: Collins.

Pereira, M. E. and C. A. McGlynn. 1997. Special relationships instead of female dominance for redfronted lemurs, *Eulemur fulvus rufus*. *American Journal of Primatology*, **43**, 239–258.

Pitman, D. 2007. *A Wild Life: Adventures of an Accidental Conservationist in Africa*. Guilford, CT: Lyons Press.

Poole, J. 1996. *Coming of Age with Elephants*. London: Hodder and Stoughton.

Port, M., D. Clough, and P. M. Kappeler. 2009. Market effects offset the reciprocation of grooming in free-ranging redfronted lemurs, *Eulemur fulvus rufus*. *Animal Behaviour*, **77**(1), 29–36.

Price, M. R. S. 1989. *Animal Re-Introductions: The Arabian Oryx in Oman*. Cambridge: Cambridge University Press.

Prins, H. H. T. 1996. *Ecology and Behaviour of the African Buffalo: Social Inequality and Decision Making*. London: Chapman and Hall.

Radford, A. N. and M. A. du Plessis. 2006. Dual function of allopreening in the cooperatively breeding green woodhoopoe, *Phoeniculus purpureus*. *Behavioral Ecology and Sociobiology*, **61**, 221–230.

Rees, L. 1997. *The Horse's Mind*. London: Ebury Press.

Reeve, H. K., D. F. Westneat, W. A. Noon, P. W. Sherman, and C. F. Aquadro. 1990. DNA fingerprinting reveals high-levels of inbreeding in colonies of the eusocial naked mole-rat. *Proceedings of the National Academy of Sciences of the United States of America*, **87**(7), 2496–2500.

Reinhardt, V. and A. Reinhardt. 1981. Cohesive relationships in a cattle herd (*Bos indicus*). *Behaviour*, **77**(3), 121–150.

Riedel, C. 2006. Prisoners rehabilitate death-row dogs. http://www.msnbc.msn.com/id/15014860/

Robbins, M. M. 1995. A demographic analysis of male life history and social structure of mountain gorillas. *Behaviour*, **132**, 21–47.

Roughgarden, J. 2004. *Evolution's Rainbow: Diversity, Gender, and Sexuality in Nature and People*. Berkeley, CA: University of California Press.

Rowlands, M. 2009. *The Philosopher and the Wolf: Lessons from the Wild on Love, Death, and Happiness*. New York: Pegasus Books.

Ryden, H. 1989. *Lily Pond: Four Years with a Family of Beavers*. New York: William Morrow.

Sapolsky, R. M. 1996. The graying of the troops. *Discover Magazine*, March 1. http://www.discovermagazine.com

Sapolsky, R. M. 2001. *A Primate's Memoir: A Neuroscientist's Unconventional Life among the Baboons*. Waterville, ME: Thorndike Press.

Schäfer, M. 1975. *The Language of the Horse: Habits and Forms of Expression*. London: Kaye and Ward.

Schaller, G. B. 1972. *The Serengeti Lion: A Study of Predator-Prey Relations*. Chicago: University of Chicago Press.

Science News. 2008. Dogs and cats can live in perfect harmony in the home if introduced in the right way. September 9. http://esciencenews.com/sources/science.daily/2008/09/09/dogs.and.cats.can.live.in.perfect.harmony.in.the.home.if.introduced.the.right.way

Scott, P. 1972. *The Swans*. London: Michael Joseph.

Sheldrick, D. 1973. *Animal Kingdom: The Story of Tsavo, the Great African Game Park*. Indianapolis: Bobbs-Merrill.

Shrader, A. M. and N. Owen-Smith. 2002. The role of companionship in the dispersal of white rhinoceroses (*Ceratotherium simum*). *Behavioral Ecology and Sociobiology*, **52**, 255–261.

Sigurjónsdóttir, H., M. C. van Dierendonck, S. Snorrason, and A. G. Thórhallsdóttir. 2003. Social relationships in a group of horses without a mature stallion. *Behaviour*, **140**, 783–804.

Sikes, S. K. 1971. *The Natural History of the African Elephant.* New York: Elsevier Publishing.

Silk, J. B. 2002. Using the 'F'-word in primatology. *Behaviour*, **139**, 421–446.

Silk, J. B., S. C. Alberts, and J. Altmann. 2003. Social bonds of female baboons enhance infant survival. *Science*, **302**, 1231–1234.

Silk, J. B., S. C. Alberts, and J. Altmann. 2006a. Social relationships among adult female baboons (*Papio cynocephalus*). II. Variation in the quality and stability of social bonds. *Behavioral Ecology and Sociobiology*, **61**, 197–204.

Silk, J. B., J. Altmann, and S. C. Alberts. 2006b. Social relationships among adult female baboons (*Papio cynocephalus*) I. Variation in the strength of social bonds. *Behavioral Ecology and Sociobiology*, **61**, 183–195.

Simpson, M. J. A. 1973. The social grooming of male chimpanzees: A study of eleven free-living males in the Gombe Stream National Park, Tanzania. In R. P. Michael and J. H. Crook, eds. *Comparative Ecology and Behaviour of Primates*, 411–505. London: Academic Press.

Skeate, S. T. 1984. Courtship and reproductive behavior of captive white-fronted Amazon parrots, *Amazona albifrons*. *Bird Behavior*, **5**, 103–109.

Slater, K. Y., C. M. Schaffner, and F. Aureli. 2009. Sex differences in the social behavior of wild spider monkeys (*Ateles geoffroyi yucatanensis*). *American Journal of Primatology*, **71**, 21–29.

Smith, D. W. and G. Ferguson. 2005. *Decade of the Wolf: Returning the Wild to Yellowstone.* Guilford, CT: Lyons Press.

Smuts, B. B. 1985. *Sex and Friendship in Baboons.* New York: Aldine Publishing.

Smuts, B. B. 2000. Battle of the sexes. In M. Bekoff, ed. *The Smile of the Dolphin*, 92–95. New York: Discovery Books.

Smuts, B. B. 2001. Encounters with animal minds. *Journal of Consciousness Studies*, **8**(5–7), 293–309.

Smuts, B. B. and J. M. Watanabe. 1990. Social relationships and ritualized greetings in adult male baboons (*Papio cynocephalus anubis*). *International Journal of Primatology*, **11**(2), 147–172.

Sommer, V. and U. Reichard. 2000. Rethinking monogamy: The gibbon case. In P. M. Kappeler, ed. *Primate Males: Causes and Consequences of Variation in Group Composition*, 159–168. Cambridge, UK: Cambridge University Press.

Stopka, P. and R. Graciasova. 2001. Conditional allogrooming in the herb-field mouse. *Behavioral Ecology*, **12**(5), 584–589.

Strier, K. B. 1992. *Faces in the Forest: The Endangered Muriqui Monkeys of Brazil.* New York: Oxford University Press.

Strier, K. B., L. T. Dib, and J. E. C. Figueira. 2002. Social dynamics of male muriquis (*Brachyteles arachnoides hypoxanthus*). *Behaviour*, **139**(2–3), 315–342.

Struhsaker, T. T. 1975. *The Red Colobus Monkey.* Chicago: University of Chicago Press.

Strum, S. C. 1987. *Almost Human: A Journey into the World of Baboons.* New York: Norton.

Stumpf, R. 2007. Chimpanzees and bonobos: Diversity within and between species. In C. J. Campbell, A. Fuentes, K. C. MacKinnon, M. Panger, and S. K. Bearder, eds. *Primates in Perspective*, 321–344. New York: Oxford University Press.

Sussman, R. W. and A. R. Chapman. 2004. *The Origins and Nature of Sociality.* New York: Aldine de Gruyter.

Sussman, R. W. and P. A. Garber. 2004. Rethinking sociality: cooperation and aggression among primates. In R. W. Sussman and A. Chapman, eds. *The Origin and Nature of Sociality*, 161–190. New York: Aldine de Gruyter.

Sussman, R. W., P. A. Garber, and J. M. Cheverud. 2005. Importance of cooperation and affiliation in the evolution of primate sociality. *American Journal of Physical Anthropology*, **128**, 84–97.

Swedell, L. 2002. Affiliation among females in wild hamadryas baboons (*Papio hamadryas hamadryas*). *International Journal of Primatology*, **23**(6), 1205–1226.

Syme, G. J. and L. A. Syme. 1979. *Social Structure in Farm Animals*. Amsterdam: Elsevier Scientific Publishing.

Takahata, Y. 1982. Social relations between adult males and females of Japanese monkeys in the Arashiyama B troop. *Primates*, **23**(1), 1–23.

Takahata, Y. 1990a. Adult males' social relations with adult females. In T. Nishida, ed. *The Chimpanzees of the Mahale Mountains: Sexual Life History Strategies*, 133–148. Tokyo: University of Tokyo.

Takahata, Y. 1990b. Social relationships among adult males. In T. Nishida, ed. *The Chimpanzees of the Mahale Mountains: Sexual Life History Strategies*, 149–170. Tokyo: University of Tokyo.

Theberge, J. [with M. T. Theberge]. 1998. *Wolf Country: Eleven Years Tracking the Algonquin Wolves*. Toronto: McClelland and Stewart.

Thomas, E. M. 1994. *The Hidden Life of Dogs*. Boston: Houghton Mifflin.

Thomas, E. M. 2009. *The Hidden Life of Deer: Lessons from the Natural World*. New York: HarperCollins.

Thouless, C. R. and F. E. Guinness. 1986. Conflict between red deer hinds: The winner always wins. *Animal Behaviour*, **34**, 1166–1171.

Tiger, L. and R. Fox. 1971. *The Imperial Animal*. New York: Holt, Rinehart, and Winston.

Trainer, J. M., D. B. McDonald, and W. A. Learn. 2002. The development of coordinated singing in cooperatively displaying long-tailed manakins. *Behavioral Ecology*, **13**(1), 65–69.

Tremain, R. 1982. *The Animals' Who's Who*. New York: Scribner's.

Turnbull-Kemp, P. 1967. *The Leopard*. London: Bailey Bros. and Swinfen.

van Hooff, J. A. R. A. M. and C. P. van Schaik. 1992. Cooperation in competition: The ecology of primate bonds. In A. H. Harcourt and F. B. M. de Waal, eds. *Coalitions and Alliances in Humans and Other Animals*, 357–389. Oxford: Oxford University Press.

van Lawick-Goodall, H. and J. van Lawick-Goodall. 1970. *Innocent Killers*. London: Collins.

van Noordwijk, M. A. and C. P. van Schaik. 2000. Reproductive patterns in eutherian mammals: adaptations against infanticide? In C. P. van Schaik and C. H. Janson, eds. *Infanticide by Males and its Implications*, 322–360. Cambridge, UK: Cambridge University Press.

van Schaik, C. P. 2000. Vulnerability to infanticide by males: patterns among mammals. In C. P. van Schaik and C. H. Janson, eds. *Infanticide by Males and its Implications*, 61–71. Cambridge, UK: Cambridge University Press.

Vavra, R. 1979. *Such is the Real Nature of Horses*. New York: Morrow.

Wahaj, S. A., N. J. Place, M. L. Weldele, S. E. Glickman, and K. E. Holekamp. 2007. Siblicide in the spotted hyena: Analysis with ultrasonic examination of wild and captive individuals. *Behavioral Ecology*, **18**(6), 974–984.

Ward, A. J. W., M. M. Webster, and P. J. B. Hart. 2007. Social recognition in wild fish populations. *Proceedings of the Royal Society B: Biological Sciences*, **274**, 1071–1077.

Watts, D. P. 1994. Social relationships of immigrant and resident female mountain gorillas, II: Relatedness, residence, and relationships between females. *American Journal of Primatology*, **32**, 13–30.

Watts, D. P. 2002. Reciprocity and interchange in the social relationships of wild male chimpanzees. *Behaviour*, **139**, 343–370.

Weber, B. and A. Vedder. 2001. *In the Kingdom of Gorillas: Fragile Species in a Dangerous Land*. New York: Simon and Schuster.

Wente, M. 2009, Feb 21. Just another member of the family? *Globe and Mail* (Toronto), A21.

Whelan, P. 1997, Jan 18. Chilly northern birders just keep on counting. *Globe and Mail* (Toronto), 18.

Whitehead, H. 2003. *Sperm Whales: Social Evolution in the Ocean*. Chicago: University of Chicago Press.

Wilkinson, G. S. 1986. Social grooming in the common vampire bat, *Desmodus rotundus*. *Animal Behaviour*, **34**(6), 1880–1889.

Williams, J. M., H. -Y. Liu, and A. E. Pusey. 2002. Costs and benefits of grouping for female chimpanzees at Gombe. In C. Boesch, G. Hohmann, and L. F. Marchant, eds. *Behavioural Diversity in Chimpanzees and Bonobos*, 192–203. Cambridge, UK: Cambridge University Press.

Woodhouse, B. 1954. *Talking to Animals 'The Woodhouse Way'*. Harmondsworth, UK: Penguin Books.

Woolfson, E. 2008. *Corvus: A Life with Birds*. London: Granta.

Wrangham, R. W. 1974. Artificial feeding of chimpanzees and baboons in their natural habitat. *Animal Behaviour*, **22**, 83–93.

Wu, H. M. H., W. G. Holmes, S. R. Medina, and G. P. Sackett. 1980. Kin preference in infant *Macaca nemestrina*. *Nature*, **285**, 225–227.

Yamagiwa, J. 1987. Intra- and inter-group interactions of an all-male group of Virunga mountain gorillas (*Gorilla gorilla beringei*). *Primates*, **28**(1), 1–30.

Young, L. C., B. J. Zaun, and E. A. VanderWerf. 2008. Successful same-sex pairing in Laysan albatross. *Biology Letters*, **4**(4), 323–325.

Zamma, K. 2002. Grooming site preferences determined by lice infection among Japanese macaques in Arashiyama. *Primates*, **43**(1), 41–49.

Zimen, E. 1981. *The Wolf: His Place in the Natural World*. London: Souvenir Press.

Notes

1. Early hunters seemed to use the "solitary" word to apply to species that could only be shot one at a time! A number of so-called solitary species are now known, after careful research using night vision equipment, radio telemetry, and molecular analysis, to be more social than once thought. Cheetahs and leopards are among these, as we shall see, as well as the small carnivore the kinkajou (*Potos flavus*) (Kays, 2003).
2. Joan Roughgarden (2004) argues that Darwin's evolutionary hypothesis of female choice (sexual selection) of a mating partner is far too simplistic and that it may never be true that a female in estrus is searching only for "a hunk with great genes."
3. There are limits to primate intelligence though. The baboon Sylvia, who was carrying her infant clutched onto her stomach, did not pause to put him on her back when she started to wade across a wide river. She walked steadily forward, apparently presuming that if her head was above water, so was that of her infant. He drowned (Cheney and Seyfarth, 2007).
4. The significance of social relationships is difficult to determine for any one species, requiring many years of research, but it can be vital. When animals, at huge expense, are re-introduced to an area that their species once inhabited, they too often fail to thrive there because of the disruption of previous social bonds between individuals, which had not been taken into account. Mark Price (1989) discovered this while working to bring Arabian oryx back to Oman. Other research shows that young pigtail macaques prefer to interact with relatives over non-relatives, even though they were raised apart from their kin including their own mother (Wu *et al.*, 1980). Therefore, friendships may be affected by relationships of which human voyeurs are unaware.
5. Although male lions have been the poster species for infanticide, female lions kill more cubs, either those of other females or their own. George Schaller (1972) documented this in his book *The Serengeti Lion*, which was published before the infanticide hypothesis was postulated and, therefore, whose data could not have been influenced by theoretical expectations as has happened since that time (Dagg, 1998, 2001). Sometimes, papers about infanticide are published and contain no knowledge of actual infant deaths, but only the idea that social structure reflects the *fear* of such deaths.
6. Although infanticide by female animals is well documented, and among rodents about as commonly inflicted by females as by males (Blumstein, 2000), scientists have expressed little interest in this topic. There has been

great excitement about chimpanzee males killing other males, aggression referred to (surely with exaggeration) as "wars," but little attention given to murderous female chimpanzees such as Passion and Pom, who were seen to snatch three infants from their mothers' arms before killing and eating them. The mother–daughter team may also have murdered seven other youngsters who disappeared from their group during the duo's infanticidal heyday (Goodall, 1986).

7. In their thoughtful article about constraints on relationships among female primates, Louise Barrett and Peter Henzi (2002) argue that perhaps there are no friendships among primates. For example, we can never know what a monkey perceives as friendship, and perhaps their cognitive capacities are incapable of this emotion in the long term. However, observations in the field show that in many if not most social species, individuals do not act randomly toward their neighbors while being sociable, but prefer to interact positively with some individuals rather than others. In this book, we consider friends to be those individuals who do interact affirmatively as has been documented by thousands of animal researchers.

8. Of course, occasionally animals provide information *because* they are captive, such as elephants that have long memories. Shirley and Jenny had once lived together at the same circus, but were then separated. When they were reunited at an Elephant Sanctuary in Tennessee 22 years later, they obviously knew each other given their frenzied greetings (Bekoff, 2002). They had remembered their friendship during all that time. As another example, observations on captive vampire bats, *Desmodus rotundus*, showed that two males liked to be together much of the time, and that some bats befriended others by regurgitating blood for them if they had not recently had a meal (DeNault and McFarlane, 1995); this type of information would be almost impossible to collect from wild bats.

IN SISTERHOOD

1. This section includes two subspecies of chimpanzees, *P. t. schweinfurthii* and *P. t. verus* from East and West Africa, respectively, which have a longer history of genetic separation than do, for example, people from Africa and China (Olson, 2006).

IN BROTHERHOOD

1. Peanuts was the first gorilla ever to touch a human, Dian Fossey (1983). Beatsme (spelled Beetsme by Fossey) was so named because Dian had no idea where he came from nor whether the animal was male or female. As early as 1975, Fossey noted that these two young gorillas were friends who traveled together.

2. Bertram (1978) notes that the high rate of copulations evolved because the females in a lion pride outnumber the males two or three to one, come into estrus quite often because of the low rate of conception, and when in heat mate frequently. He calculates that during his lifetime a successful pride male would copulate about 20,000 times.

MOTHERS AND DAUGHTERS

1. Sociobiologists believe that the evolutionary reason for a youngster to try to delay its mother's next conception is because when the mother produces a new infant, this event will reduce her care and support for this youngster, to its disadvantage (Ghiglieri, 1988).

2. Harcourt does not identify the gorillas involved in his study either by name or number. This is unfortunate because the reader cannot use his data to increase their knowledge about the same individuals named and described in detail by Dian Fossey and other researchers. Reading his article today makes it seem that animals are not important for themselves, but only for obtaining generalizations about primate behavior. Yet only by knowing more about individuals can we acquire more nuanced information. In addition, it now seems more vital than ever to have readers empathize with animals by giving them names, to help activists fight against the extinction of whole species.

There has been much discussion about how to identify individual animals in a field study. Early researchers such as Jane Goodall (1986) and Elizabeth Marshall Thomas (1994) were told not to use names for animals lest their work seem unscientific. Goodall further notes that when she submitted her first research paper for publication, it was returned from a major academic journal with the pronouns "he," "she," and "who" crossed out and the words "it" and "which" substituted. (That a qualified reviewer in the 1960s believed it did not matter if an animal were male or female shows what a long way we have come in the study of animal behavior since then!) As recently as 1981, the anthropologist Colin Turnbull refused to give a favorable endorsement to Fossey's book *Gorillas in the Mist* because she had given the animals names rather than numbers (Montgomery, 1991). Cynthia Moss reports (1988) that some scientists thought that using names for individual animals was taboo because a researcher might associate one of them with a person he or she knew with the same name, and impose that person's characteristics onto the animal. (Of course, because she spent so much time with her elephants, Moss might have associated an elephant's characteristics with one of her human friends if it had the same name, although this would not bother the elephant.) All of these women scientists repudiated such concerns and used names for individuals (as I did for giraffe in my 1950s field study) because names seemed more humane and were easier to remember than numbers. Perhaps in part to address Moss's concern (although he writes that he actually likes Biblical appellations), Robert Sapolski (2001) gave his animals Old Testament names such as Solomon, Josiah, and Naomi.

By contrast, John Theberge (1998) chose to identify the wolves he studied in Algonquin Park, Ontario by the names of lakes in their territories in order that he did *not* humanize them. The men who numbered rather than named the 31 collared wolves brought from Canada to reoccupy Yellowstone National Park in 1995 and 1996 were said by their wives to have done so because they feared that some of the wolves would not survive. They felt that this loss would be more tolerable if the wolf had a number rather than a name. Tim Clutton-Brock (2007) officially identified his 300 known meerkats with code numbers, but he and his associates in the field often used whimsical names that were easy to remember for these same individuals. Wild animals studied by behaviorists would not know if they had a name or number in the records, but perhaps the scientists who named rather than numbered them came across to the animals as more empathetic? Might this perception be reflected in the data they collected?

Thinking about the importance of names, British scientists Catherine Douglas and Peter Rowlinson (2009) from Newcastle University wondered if naming a cow would influence the amount of milk she produced. When they asked 516 U.K. dairy farmers about this question, 46 percent agreed that naming must make a difference because, on average, those with names produced 258 more liters of milk a year compared to unnamed cows. Sixty percent of the farmers said that they knew all the cows in their herd, while 48 percent agreed that positive human contact was likely to produce cows with a good milking temperament. The researchers conclude that "Placing more importance on knowing the individual animals and calling them by name can – at no extra cost to the farmer – also significantly increase milk production." Playing classical (not modern) music in the milking barn and handling the cows gently also increases milk production (Hatkoff, 2009).

FATHERS AND SONS, AND SOCIAL GROOMING AND PREENING

1. Banjo disappeared when he was six months old. Fossey did not know what had happened to him, so she decided to collect the dung from each of the nests that the individual gorillas had made at night, and then analyze the feces to see if they contained remnants of the infant. They did this by straining each turd in the creek near her camp, hunting for tiny fragments of infant bone or hair. They found these in the stools of Effie and her daughter Puck, but not in those of Icarus.

FAMILY AND GROUP TIGHT BONDS

1. Irven Buss (1990) was hired to study (and destroy) the elephants in the name of science. When he and a colleague noticed a relationship among three adult females and a young calf, they decided to shoot the two younger females first to see what the old matriarch would do. At their deaths, she rushed frantically to one of the females followed by her calf, who fell into a hole behind her, so she then sped back to him, trying frantically to dig him out. "Excitement and stress stimulated activation of her temporal glands, which were now secreting rather copiously," Buss noted. Fearing the mother would bury her infant by mistake, they shot her too (becoming no. 47 in their collection), and then her calf (becoming no. 48). Buss was pleased to send nearly three tons of "material" back to Washington State University where he was a professor.
2. In the Pacific coastal waters of British Columbia and Washington State, orcas, which have been closely studied for decades, occur in two distinct races. The resident race described here consumes migratory salmon and other fish (Knudtson, 1996). Its members apparently do not interbreed with members of the transient race who feed on seals, sea lions, and dolphins; they have a larger geographic range but lack long-lasting stable families and sophisticated vocalizations.
3. The scientific name of this species is somewhat in flux (Theberge, 1998). The Algonquin animals initially were thought to be gray wolves (*Canis lupus*) until DNA analysis indicated that they were probably red wolves (*Canis rufus*), which have become largely extinct in eastern North America. It may be that they should be called *Canis lycaon*, the eastern timber wolf. The confusion is

compounded by some interbreeding of the Algonquin wolves with coyotes (*Canis latrans*).
4. Chimpanzees and crows have brains that are about the same size relative to their body weights, but crows can use tools better than can chimpanzees (*A Murder of Crows*, 2009).

SOCIAL BUT SELDOM SOCIABLE ANIMALS

1. Meredith Bashaw watched a herd of 12 Rothschild's giraffe in the Wild Animal Park of San Diego Zoo for 18 months (Milius, 2003). She discovered that some individuals, who of course had limited space in which to wander, were more likely than others to be close together: some dyads spent, at most, 15 percent of the time together, while others hobnobbed for only a third as long.

   At the Marwell Wildlife Zoo in England where animals have much less room to move about, Paul Rose (2010) documented, over a three-year period, possible associations among giraffe in a herd of seven to 11 animals. He defined associations as individuals within one neck length of each other who were standing, lying, or grooming. He did not include feeding "as this stimulus over-rode the desire to seek out a specific partner." His work is on-going, but he has found that Matilda and Isabella were more likely to be near each other than to be near any other giraffe.

2. Wildlife researchers usually assume that capturing, anesthetizing, and fixing tags or collars on wild animals does them no harm. In their careful study, however, Festa-Bianchet and Côté (2008) found to their horror that mountain goats were very sensitive to being handled by people. First, they realized on checking their results that a mother who had been captured and drugged was more likely than other mothers to abandon her kid. So they stopped handling nursing nannies. Then they found that kids who had been captured were less likely to be seen again than other kids and may have died, so they stopped capturing kids. Two other problems were that, in some years, kids with radio collars were less likely to survive than kids with ear tags, and that young females caught and drugged were less likely than other young females to produce a kid the following year. Most studies of ungulates being drugged and handled have had at least some undesirable consequences, but perhaps none were as serious as those suffered by the mountain goats (Côté *et al.*, 1998).

   Research on birds may have negative repercussions too. In his study of the grey-faced petrel, Mike Imber (1976) dug openings of about half a meter (1.6 ft) from each of many burrows so that the occupants could be observed (with the help of a mirror and torch light), caught, banded, and have their weight and bill measurements recorded. He tried to minimize harm to the birds, but even so, he reports that apparently, because of handling or observation, up to 10 percent of pairs deserted their burrows, had their eggs broken, and often their pair-bonds permanently destroyed as well.

   Festa-Bianchet and Côté (2008) insist that it is no longer acceptable to assume that manipulations of individual wild animals have no adverse effects on them and their population. Such procedures are unethical and, if at all negative for the animals, will produce flawed results.

3. When I went to Africa in 1956 to study the behavior of giraffe, for lack of all other such field studies Darling's *A Herd of Red Deer* was the only book

recommended to me as a guide on how to proceed, even though it had been written twenty years earlier. This indicates how recent is the discipline of ethology, research on the behavior of animals in their natural habitats.

ANIMAL AND HUMAN "FRIENDSHIPS"

1. Stanley Coren (2010) speculates that the close association of people and dogs over thousands of years has shaped the behavior and evolution of people as well as of dogs. Dogs are more likely to risk their lives helping a human companion in danger if he or she has been kind to them; in consequence, such a caring person will be more likely to live longer. Thus, a dog's heroism toward people increases the probability of human compassion toward dogs in the future. A canine hero will be well treated with good food and protection, so that dog heroism may benefit both the hero and his or her future progeny.

2. Even reptiles can have preferred friends. Dr Lee Harding (personal communication, March 2010) writes that his son Andrew kept lizards of various species as pets over the years, which were allowed to roam around a room at times. One of them was comfortable with family members, but if a strange person, reptile, or dog came through the door, it immediately fled to Andrew, ran up his body and cringed against his head, on the side away from the intruder. In times of danger, it did not flee to a dark corner or to its terrarium, but to its buddy Andrew.

3. As another viewpoint on Washoe, Vicki Hearne in her book *Adam's Task* (2000) describes a walk that the chimpanzee took with Fouts and a friend, which entailed "the use of leashes, a tiger hook and a cattle prod," just in case. She was told that she could watch this outing, but only from a distance and if she kept very still. She wonders if there can be a real friendship between two individuals when their status is so unequal. Hearne also believes that dogs and horses have a language sense (in the meaning of being able to communicate with another being) that far exceeds that of any chimpanzee.

4. If Nim could have communicated his thoughts, what might they have been? One psycholinguist imagined that he would demand "a quarter to call his lawyer to get him out of this joint" (Hess, 2008). A historian suggested, "If we could hear them speak, we might not want to hear what they say." Surely an understatement.

Index